CHI KUNG BREATHING EXERCISES FOR HEALTH, RELAXATION AND ENERGY

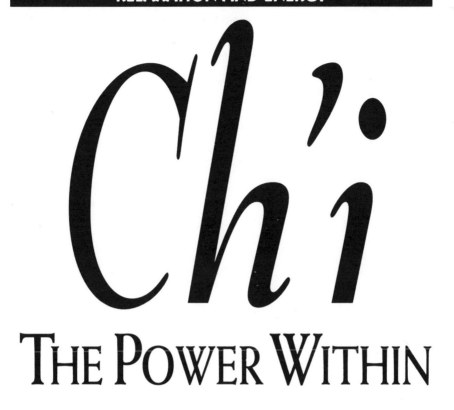

Ch'i

THE POWER WITHIN

GEOFF PIKE
& PHYLLIS PIKE

TUTTLE PUBLISHING
Boston · Rutland, Vermont · Tokyo

DEDICATION
FOR DR. B. M. KOTEWALL, whose help and support is unfailing.

A NOTE OF CAUTION: Before beginning this, or any other, exercise program, it is advisable to obtain the approval and recommendation of your physician. While you are on this or any exercise program, it is advisable to visit your physician for periodic monitoring. The information in this book is intended to supplement, and not replace, treatment by a physician or other licensed medical practitioner. The adoption and application of the information in this book is at the readers discretion and sole responsibility. the author and publisher of this book are not responsible in any manner whatsoever for any injury that may occur indirectly or directly from the use of this book.

First published in the United States of America in 1996 by Charles E. Tuttle Co., Inc. of Rutland, Vermont, and Tokyo, Japan, with editorial offices at 153 Milk Street, Boston, Massachusetts, 02109.

Library of Congress Catalog Card Number: 96-042110
ISBN 0-8048-3099-1

Distributed by:

North America, Latin America & Europe
Tuttle Publishing
Distribution Center
Airport Industrial Park
364 Innovation Drive
North Clarendon, VT 05759-9436
Tel: (802) 773-8930
Fax: (802) 773-6993
Email: info@tuttlepublishing.com

Asia Pacific
Berkeley Books Pte Ltd
130 Joo Seng Road
#06-01/03 Olivine Building
Singapore 368357
Tel: (65) 6280-1330
Fax: (65) 6280-6290
Email: tuttle-sales@gol.com

Japan
Tuttle Publishing
Yaekari Bldg., 3F
5-4-12 Ōsaki, Shinagawa-ku
Tokyo 141 0032
Tel: (03) 5437-0171
Fax: (03) 5437-0755
Email: inquiries@periplus.com.sg

06 05 04 03   10 9 8 7 6 5 4 3

Printed in the United States of America

AUTHOR'S NOTE

It is almost 20 years since I was first introduced to these ancient Chinese breathing exercises — behind the crumbling walls of the Escolta — Manila's Old China Town. Their regular practice helped me through the most difficult and dangerous period of my life and continue to play an important part in my everyday exercise routine.

When they were first published in 1980 under the title *The Power of Ch'i*, I was satisfied that I had at least tried to share their remarkable benefits with others interested in self help and self discovery. I did not dream that *The Power of Ch'i* would quickly become an international best-seller and that tens of thousands of people would be practising Pa Tuan Tsin — The Eight Precious Sets of Exercises — for health and longevity.

Since then the book has been reprinted each year and the number of its practitioners has become countless as has the numbers of letters received from all over the world. The renaissance of Therapeutic Chi Kung (Restorative Breathing Exercises) has spread throughout China as a daily fitness program, a vital part of preventative medicine, a regenerative program for the ageing and in many cases, relief and cure of degenerative and malignant disease.

In Western society and in Western medical science, attitudes towards health and fitness have also changed over the past 13 years. Aspects of traditional Chinese medicine that were once ignored or frowned upon are becoming more and more accepted and practised.

The fitness industry now encompasses physical culture centres, sports medicine consultants, nutritionists, health foods, modern exercise equipment, health and fitness magazines and a growing number of books on wellbeing and self development.

All of these go hand in hand with naturopathy, herbal medicine, acupuncture, Oriental massage, meditation, relaxation techniques and an increasing interest in authentic martial arts. In *Ch'i: The Power Within* you will find a reasonably simple combination of the old and the new: ancient breathing exercises combined with compatible Western health methods that if followed with a gentle determination for approximately 30 minutes a day will greatly improve your physical and mental harmony. Above all else be patient with your progress, tolerant of your body and mind, as disciplined as possible in your practice and check with your doctor if you have any respiratory or spinal ailments.

Geoff Pike

CONTENTS

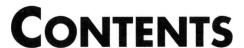

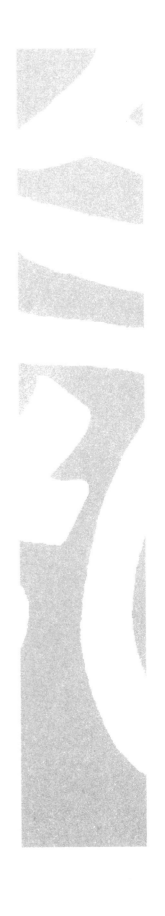

INTRODUCTION

In 1975, while living in the Philippines, I was found to have cancer. Today, at the age of sixty-four, I am fit, healthy and a great believer in the breathing exercises I have demonstrated in this book. I have no way of proving how much their daily practice had to do with my recovery but I do know that they have given me a new outlook and renewed vitality.

The shock of this news came at a time when I had reached a robust middle age and was enjoying the fruits of a successful career, an exciting if somewhat vagabond lifestyle and a tranquil marriage that gave me everything to live for. It caused me to look back at my life and wonder where, when, why and how I had first yielded to this awful disease. The inexplicable carcinoma that modern science seems powerless to fathom, this disorderly ganging up of cells, strikes a dread as great as any human or inhuman threat. Yet we live with it every day of our lives, ignoring its victims unless they are close to us and even avoiding the very word that describes it. There is nothing else to be done. It is something, we feel sure, that is set aside for others, never for us.

Perhaps it is this terrible feeling of loneliness, this helplessness of being singled out for the worst of all punishments, that makes one take stock. It is amazing how quickly a lifetime can shrink and how insignificant its purpose can become. One thing, however, that must shine through is the realisation that we alone are responsible for our bodies and their continued performance. Our care or neglect and our knowledge of our physical and mental make-up can do much to decide the state of health we enjoy or endure, especially in later years.

If you are to take any notice of this book and follow its suggestions at all, you should probably know something about its author and the life he has led. This is an outline of the life I was forced to look back on when threatened with the possibility of its untimely end.

I was born in Edmonton, London, in 1929. My early childhood was spent in Waltham Cross, Hertfordshire, where my father managed an off-licence liquor store. He was slowly dying as a result of too many months in the front-line trenches of Verdun and the

Somme. Once he had been a gymnast and singer of note. Now, twenty years later, his lungs had all but collapsed and disease ran riot through his body and mind. I can remember the awful lassitude that took hold of him, a terrible, lonely anguish that left him less and less active. I was probably seven or eight years old when I vowed that such a thing would never be allowed to happen to me.

Circumstance and the Second World War then gave me a couple of enchanting years as an evacuee in the Essex countryside before I was admitted to a naval training ship. Harsh treatment, harsher food and hard work in bitter Welsh weather seemed to do me no harm, and by the time I went to sea at the age of fifteen and seven months, I had learned to smoke and drink and was more than ready to grapple with the world.

My first great shock came on my sixteenth birthday. Stepping ashore in Kure, Japan, I took the train to Hiroshima. It was only a month or two after the atomic bomb had been dropped and what I saw and felt is still indescribable. Most astonishing of all was the sight of an old Japanese man standing among the ruins of what must have been his home and practising his breathing exercises.

I was to see more of this mysterious discipline in India and among the Chinese of Singapore and Indo-China. Each morning in the ports of Bombay and Calcutta there were those who would come down to the waterfront to exercise. It was in Saigon that I first saw a demonstration of the Chinese martial arts and the ancient breathing exercises that make its mastery possible.

After a year or so aboard an oil tanker in the Persian Gulf, I jumped ship in Sydney and went inland in search of trees. Trees are a thing you miss at sea. I drifted wherever opportunity took me. The outback of mid-western New South Wales showed me the inside of sheep station bunkhouses, shearing sheds, railway fettlers' tents, sawmills and drovers' camps. The food was always rough but plentiful, work was hard and the drinking of beer in monumental quantities was an essential part of bush existence.

After two eventful and fascinating years, I was ready again for the smell of the sea and eventually went back to England where I was conscripted to the Royal Artillery.

Demobbed in 1954, I returned to Australia, took a job in a warehouse and began studying art at night school. By 1960, I had become a respectable married man with all the accumulations of moderate success. My taste for plain and simple food was still with me, as was my capacity for beer and cigarettes. The need for physical work (for mine was the desk-bound job of a director of animated films) I fulfilled with half-hearted attempts at weight-training.

It was not until 1967 that I again came into contact with the Orient that had so impressed me as a boy. Now creative director of an advertising agency in Hong Kong, I used to walk each morning through Victoria Park or the villages of the New Territories and watch the Chinese of all ages and walks of life practising the same kinds of exercises I had seen twenty years earlier.

My interest grew and for the next six years I travelled extensively in Southeast Asian countries to delve further into Oriental myth and legend, folklore and traditional attitudes towards health, healing and longevity.

BEFORE WE BEGIN

If your inner strength is matched only by your quietude of mind, then you are either too young to read this book, or this is not your particular mountain.

Are you one of those rare beings who consistently conducts a satisfactory life in good order and with reasonable success, effectively managing your mental and physical capabilities with sensible discipline? Have you learned with patience and foresight to nurture your health and treasure your one and only body with humility and gratitude?

Have you at all times avoided excess, never overindulged your appetites and senses, maintained with fortitude and determination your precious youth, beginning each day with renewed zest and ending it in sound, untroubled sleep?

Is your sex life garlanded with sensual security, unhindered by inhibitions, haemorrhoids or hernia? Are you unaware and undisturbed by your joints, nerves, anxieties, the threats of war, pollution, disease, ageing, God Almighty and inevitable death?

Do your bowels move with the regularity of the rising and setting of the sun? Do you have a digestive system as dependable as the ebb and flow of the tide? Does the temperature and rhythm of your blood waver only when it should? Do the freedom of your movements, brightness of your eye and the bloom upon your skin bring glances of envy and admiration?

If you can say yes to all these conditions then you also probably do not need to read further. On the other hand, if you are an average specimen of twentieth-century humanity, pronounced 'fit' by your general practitioner but knowing you could feel better, please read on.

It does not matter whether the realisation that you are 'not feeling as well as you should be', that you are 'not getting any younger' occurs to you in circumstances exotic or mundane. It could be under a guava tree on a Filipino hilltop as it was for me, behind a desk or a lawn mower, in bed alone or with someone else, running for the bus or just walking the dog. Neither does it matter what age you may be or the condition you are in. This book is not written for the middle-aged, but rather for those who feel middle-aged or know that some day they will.

What does matter is that we are all, without exception, dependent upon one thing, air: oxygen is the one and only essential available to all human beings in equal shares, to be used as we see fit. Breath gives life, sustains it and takes it away. Without it, we weaken, sicken and expire; because of it, we are revived, refreshed and quickly restored.

As with most things freely available and known to be good for us, we tend to take the important business of breathing for granted. The simple process of inhalation and exhalation need hardly be considered. Our supply of air is always constant and there is plenty of it. Only when it is threatened with pollution or infiltrated by unwelcome odours, do we become aware of it or indignant about our right to breathe it. Only when our breathing is impaired by age or ill health, do we show concern.

When we are fortunate enough to find ourselves on a mountain or close to the open sea, we fill our laboured lungs like nomads at an oasis, muttering things like 'absolute tonic … air like wine … feel it doing you good … glad to be alive'. And then, after a few hasty gulps, we return to our daily grind where the last thing we think of is deep breathing.

The Asians have known the importance of breath control for thousands of years. It is no coincidence that the great yogis and sadhus of India, the lamas of Tibet, the holy men and sages of China automatically took to mountainous regions for meditation and self-development or that all of their achievements, both physical and spiritual, began and ended with the harnessing of the air around them and its channelling into remarkable powers.

Unfortunately, access to mountain tops and the salty broads of oceans is becoming more and more restricted in the daily life of the average person. The promise of this book is to explain and demonstrate the truly amazing health benefits to be drawn from the air that surrounds you, whatever your location and whatever your circumstances.

WHAT IS CH'I?

What is this miraculous thing called Ch'i, this power that can rehabilitate failing health and recharge the human spirit, arrest illness and keep disease at bay? Can Ch'i really prolong vigorous life, regain lost years? Where did it come from? How can I find this key to the shining health, expanding energy and sheer physical joy I enjoyed briefly as a child? I had it then. Is it really possible that I can have it again? And, if I find it, how can I possibly hold onto it for the rest of my days?

To define Ch'i in simple terms one would have to know more than the yogis of India, the lamas of Tibet, the Shinto priests of Japan and the ancient sages of China. For at least five millennia wise people of the East have known its secret, but have been unable or unwilling to share it. The yogi calls it *Prana*, the lama calls it *Lung-gom*; to the follower of Shinto it is *Sakia-tundra* or *ki*, to the Chinese it is Ch'i. All seek the same source and all reach the same summit, as clear and immovable as a mountain on a diamond-bright day, as steady and changeless as that seat of meditation, the Himalayas. It is perhaps best described in the following passage from *The Secret of The Golden Flower: A Chinese Book of Life* (trans. Richard Wilhelm, Harvest Books, New York, 1970):

> *Heaven created water through the One. That is the true energy of the great One. If man attains the One he becomes alive; if he loses it he dies. But even if man lives in the energy (vital breath) he does not see the energy, just as fishes live in water but do not see the water. Man dies when he has not vital breath, just as fishes perish when deprived of water. If one guards this true energy, one can prolong the span of life and can apply the method of creating an immortal body.*

Two other well known students of the Eastern occult comment on the importance of breathing to longevity. Under the heading of 'Exercises for Prolonging Life', in *Chinese Folk Medicine* (Mentor Books, USA, 1974) Heinrich Wallnofer and Anna von Rottauscher state:

> *Correct breathing is the basis of all exercises recommended in China for longevity, as well as for the cure of several diseases. As early as the*

fourth century BC, the philosopher Chuang-tzu promulgated that men of great wisdom fetch their breath from deep inside and below, while ordinary men breathe with the larynx alone. In other words, men were even then aware of the great value of deep respiration.

The principal purpose of Chinese gymnastic exercises, as is the purpose of the Indian yoga practices, is to attain proper circulation of the blood which, in turn, will ensure emotional balance and stability. This stability is to lend the body resistance against illnesses and consequently grant a longer healthier life. Correct breathing is also mentioned very early as a means of cleansing the blood and body of their debris. Congestions may be removed and stiff joints limbered by adhering to the pertinent exercise instructions.

Contrary to many yoga practices, Chinese exercises are quite simple throughout and demand neither particular exertion, nor extraordinary and violent bodily contortions. Still, perseverance and strong willpower are indispensable if one wants to attain the final goal. All details are prescribed minutely, from the body posture to the exact position and motion of the fingers, and they have to be followed methodically.

Surely, you say, such a blessing as Ch'i must be available to only a gifted few? On the contrary it is available to every man, woman and child, rich or poor, regardless of age, colour or creed. It is always there, awaiting those with the determination to reach for it. It surrounds us wherever we are. It is presented to us all at birth. We can use it as we please, cherish or waste it as we see fit. It is as close as our next breath or as distant as the horizon: the first gift given, the first lesson learned, and the last to be taken away.

I will never know how much the ancient exercises contained in this book had to do with my recovery from cancer, how much was due to 'super-voltage', my 'Maker', Ch'i, or a combination of all three. I am certain, though, that the continual daily practice of *The Eight Precious Sets of Exercises*, known to the Chinese as *Pa Tuan Tsin*, fortified me against the ravages of massive radiation and proved invaluable during recuperation. This opinion was shared by Dr Robert Morrison, Director of Radiation Therapy at Hammersmith Hospital in England.

Ch'i can be cultivated by learning the breathing exercises contained in this book. It can be developed by practising them for a short period of time each day, in place of, or as well as, any exercise routine you may already have adopted. It costs nothing, requires no equipment or training partner … just air to breathe and room to move. You can develop the power of Ch'i to whatever degree your patience and personal fortitude will allow and retain it for the rest of your life.

FACING THE CONDITION YOU ARE IN

*Rolled around in earth's diurnal course
with rocks and stones and trees.*

William Wordsworth

PART ONE

THE HILL

If you can believe the people you meet and talk to on the subject, or perhaps your own friends, whom you have watched as they grow older, it seems that middle age and the decline of physical condition creep up on some people quite comfortably while others are hit as though with a club. The exceptions are usually very active individuals who either have the circumstances to allow a physically active lifestyle or a continuing dedication to some kind of sport.

We have all admired the professional ski instructor, swimming, tennis or football coach; the golf pro or gym instructor who is well past forty and still going strong. Consider the people who have spent a lifetime outdoors engaged in some kind of physical work. Chances are, they are stronger and sounder than their counterpart behind a desk, closeted in air-conditioning and artificial light. It stands to reason that the active outdoor types who use their bodies continually stand a better chance of a long and healthy life than those who think for a living and let their bodies go to waste. In the computerised 1990s, with physical effort becoming increasingly unpopular, it's not surprising that even something as obvious as this can become obscured by the daily round of survival.

It is true that people in the West are becoming more aware of their responsibility for their own physical and mental welfare. There is less and less excuse for poor condition: we have increased leisure time, sporting and fitness centres, swimming pools, home gymnasium equipment, diet charts, health foods, nature cures, vitamins and all the advice and encouragement one can ask for in self-help books and mass media programs. Many people take advantage of these opportunities and maintain a steady keep-fit routine throughout their lives but many others simply let themselves go and hope for the best.

For most of us the simple business of keeping body and soul in one piece, being responsible for a family, a home and a career is all we can cope with. We are 'kept going' by the sheer momentum of necessity, whether in a unionised work-force or on different levels of personal endeavour and ambition. It is often only in middle years, when vital energy begins to show a little wear, that it occurs to us that we may not be immortal. Our precious youth is all but spent because it probably has not been well maintained. Many of us have squandered it, taking fitness and health for granted and then wondering, quite suddenly, where it has gone. Is it too late to get it back? Health and strength came so naturally a few years ago ... now it may take effort and discipline. We know it is worth it, but how?

The story that follows is how it happened for me — how I came to face the shape I was in and what I did about it. I have tried to give as accurate an account as possible, and because this was undoubtedly the turning point of my life it is not difficult to remember.

The road to Taal Volcano wanders out from 'metro' Manila with the aimlessness of a lost buffalo and heads for the hills. It leaves the clutter of the outer barrios (slums) and the tangle of traffic. It straightens out between the rice paddies that flow, as if infinite, towards Batangas and the Sibuyan Sea. The landscape becomes prettier as you climb higher: sugar cane, pineapple and coconut groves. Villages are few and far between: clean, earth yards well swept; bougainvillea and wild banana shading the grass thatch. Dusty chickens and muddy pigs scatter as you drive through. The people grin. As in most countries, they get happier and friendlier the further you get from the city.

I was travelling in the company's air-conditioned, chauffeur-driven Chevrolet to a seminar at Taal. The company thought the mist-shrouded majesty of the volcano and its sapphire lake was a suitable background for the business at hand and therefore worth the two-and-a-half-hour drive. We were an hour out when the front offside tyre blew, right in the middle of nowhere.

It was a hot day. It was hot all over. The earth was hot, the grass, the trees, the bushes, stones, sprouts, shoots, everything was hot. Even the birds hid among toasted leaves. Everything that stood, grew, flew or just lay around and burned was oppressed by the heat. Consumed by it. I was hottest of all. I wondered if I would have felt as afflicted by it had I been ten years younger. I tried to remember. I couldn't. I was too damn hot to think.

Maybe that was why I decided to climb the hill. It could be cooler up there. It wasn't! A single guava tree sheltered its peak like a peasant's hat. Its shade was sauna-hot. I looked down to where the car baked, a silver shell in the smothering shade of bamboo that cracked like stones in a fire and rustled dead leaves under the shrilling weight of cicadas.

That car was something special. The kind we all watch going by when we were on the way up and dreamed of owning when we made it to where we were going. Right now, it looked about as impressive as the tin can I used to kick down gutters. The jacket I carried was pretty special too. Tropical fabric, carefully chosen from an expensive wad of muted shades, in the best available taste. Hand-cut, styled and stitched by costly artisan's fingers, just for me. Up here, it felt like a wet sugar sack.

I should have felt great in that great suit, looking back at that great car. I didn't. I felt sick. I felt strung out. I felt like an old man in a young man's pants. Insects whirred and clacked in the leaves over my aching skull. The cool green skin of a guava fruit showed, just out of reach. Did you know the inside of a guava stays cool like a melon, even in this equatorial intensity? I tried for one. Stretched and made an attempt to jump. It was like reaching for the hand of God. Sweat, not perspiration. Plain, salty sweat ran down the inside of that special suit the way rain runs down a roof in a monsoon. The only heart I'll ever own beat like a Salvation Army drum on a sunny Sabbath. Blood churned around, a mill-race in my ears. A heart attack? After taking on one lousy little hill?

Knees of guava jelly. I sat. The rock was hot, so I stood. A short pull at the silver hip flask, encased in Spanish leather and monogrammed in gold. The best of Scottish malt to the rescue. The cigarette I lit, selected from a flat gold case, was the brand of smoke expected of successful executives, to be lit with a gold Dunhill. Sucking back the smoke and looking at my solid gold watch. You know the kind of watch it was? Right! A Rolex. Hewn from a solid ingot, the ad said. I had it all. Man, was I successful! But I couldn't reach a guava, or climb a tree to save my sensational life!

So there I am. Reviewing my life from the top of this piddling hill. Have you ever done that? Not necessarily from a Filipino hilltop, maybe from your office window, or on the beach, holding your stomach in. In the bath with everything out of sight but a belly-button full of suds. A popular place for quiet analysis is the sanctuary of the bathroom, wondering why things don't work the way they used to. It's a great place to come to terms with your hair, teeth and overall shape.

Anyway, right now, back to me, and my unattainable guava. I was pretty successful in business. Not a tycoon or anything like that, but pretty well set-up in a self-made, independent sort of way. The company car, the driver, the wardrobe, the heavy trinkets, the five-star hotels, monumental menus, fat expense account and first-class air fares all went along with fat fees. Mine was a pretty sought-after existence. A consultant in the worldwide business of 'Creative Communications'.

Usually, it's called advertising. But when you've been at it as long as I have, you like to think of it as communication. That's when you've sold just about all there is to sell, from peanuts to computers, to just about all the people there are in your share of the world and somebody else's share; sold soft drinks where they need water, and chocolate where they need medicine; and learned about likes and dislikes, market reactions and motivations. When you have used the Big Brother tactics of market research and consumer analysis to manipulate minds with purchase propositions, persuasion, penetration, test targets and creative strategies, then you like to think of it as communication. But really, it is advertising. What we do for a living doesn't matter either. We're getting older every day. Maybe more or less successful, but older. What are we doing about it? That's what matters!

So, that was my particular concern around the time I realised I was becoming a physical failure. I had reached the top of my professional tree. Trouble-shooting for international advertising agencies over half the world, in particular the Eastern half, but I could have been washing cars in Baltimore or seeding salmon in the Scottish Highlands. It wouldn't have made any difference. I had used up the first half of my life. I had squandered it like a pirate digging into a chest of silver. I was looking at the bottom. Where had it all gone? I try to think back over the scattered years, to when I could have raced down that hill and up again without breathing hard.

Youth. I remember mine. It probably wasn't anything at all like yours. Then again, maybe it was in some ways. For one thing, we both took it for granted. Because we never ached or strained or sprained. Middle age was something that happened to other people, like getting hit by a bus. We were immortal. Remember? Age was always five years ahead of us.

Midday. Hairs on my wrist stuck flat and moisture under the glass of the fabulous Rolex Oyster. I was going to be late. I wondered if my driver felt this blast furnace, black as a beetle around that front wheel. He moved slowly as do many Filipinos. Well-defined muscles, under that uniform shirt he'd shed, rolled with his efforts the way mine once rolled.

SOME SIMPLE TESTS

So that's how it happened for me. Of course, these little moments of truth pass and we feel 'quite all right' again. We bury them quickly. We may be so unaccustomed to exercise that our make-up soon settles down to its indolent routine and we get along perfectly well, until the next time. And there will be a next time unless, of course, we eventually fall ill or have an accident from which an unfit body cannot recover. You don't have to climb a hill without a hat in 100 degrees and 100 per cent humidity to feel like dropping out of the big parade. You can let your guard down, lower your defences, get a little afraid, a little tired of it all any time and anywhere. But sooner or later, it will happen. So don't wait. If you want to get some idea of the kind of shape you are in there are a couple of very simple tests you can try right now, in the office, the kitchen, the bathroom, the garden, anywhere but a phone booth. All you need is room enough to breathe, spread your arms, jump 15 centimetres and bend double.

First the lungs. Try taking three very long, deep breaths, inhaling through the nose as slowly and silently as you can. Hold each breath for the count of three, exhale through the mouth as slowly and silently as you can and again count to three before taking the next breath. It is likely that you'll find the inhalation shortish and somehow unsatisfactory, like only finding the capacity to drink half a glass of water when you're thirsty. You may find the exhalation hard to control, as though your lungs are unaccustomed to overfilling and eager to spill out.

Average lungs don't like to be reminded that they are only working at half their capacity, even if they feel overworked. You may experience brief dizziness, possibly fleeting patterns before your eyes. You will almost certainly feel strange in some way if you really tried to fill your normally half-filled lungs, especially if you are a smoker.

Before considering concentrated breathing of any kind, it is vitally important to 'build up to it'. The fact that you have been breathing all your life doesn't immediately qualify you for intense breathing exercises. Look at it this way: you have been walking all your life, but you would soon drop out of a marathon; you have been lifting things all your life, but you would be unwise to attempt lifting a 100 kilogram weight; you may have been swimming since you were a child, but could you swim 8 kilometres to shore?

Most 'normal' breathers would find it distinctly uncomfortable, even painful, to suddenly begin filling their lungs to four or five times their usual capacity. Your system just isn't used to taking in that much oxygen at once. Fuel of life or not, you can overfill your tank too suddenly. The trick is to clean it out and make it larger for a start. Unless you are already well practised in deep breathing, the best thing you can do is to set this book aside when you have read it, for a week or a month or whatever it takes to build up your lung power.

Begin practising deep breathing whenever and wherever it occurs to you to do so. While walking, resting, working or even preparing for sleep. Make regular, conscious efforts to increase your breath load. During this process your ribcage will expand and with it, the ease and capacity of your respiration. You may find that you gain up to 2 centimetres around the chest. In a month's time, it may have expanded another 2 centimetres or even more to the full extent your frame will allow. In the first six months of conscious breathing my own chest expansion went from 97 to 105 to 113 centimetres; in the second six months from 113 to 116 to 120 centimetres.

Now that you have found that your breathing techniques could use a little attention, let's get to the flexibility of waist, neck, arms and legs. If you're in normal health and over thirty — that is to say, you don't plough fields, chop trees, demolish buildings or re-sleeper railway lines for a living — you have probably lost your flexibility.

There are some simple tests for flexibility of neck, legs and arms that you can try on the spot. First the neck: stand erect, rise on your toes and slowly try looking behind you without swivelling your shoulders. Try this three times to the left and three times to the right. You'll probably find you can't get far without risk of breaking something. After six weeks of Pa Tuan Tsin, you will think you are made of India rubber.

Next, the legs. Stand erect, with heels together. Inhale deeply and slowly. Lower your body gradually, exhaling as you go down until you are squatting in a deep knee bend. Do not touch the floor with your fingers. Count to three and try slowly standing up. If you can do this three times without drums beating in your ears and your kneecaps going off like toy pistols, try another three. Probably, you will find it hard to rise steadily on the first attempt: almost impossible on the second and very difficult on the third. After six weeks of Pa Tuan Tsin you will be bobbing up and down as easily as a well-greased, fiddler's elbow.

Lastly, the arms and shoulders. Stretch them out to their full extent, locking the elbows and force them back at shoulder level. See how far behind you can reach without threat of dislocation or springing a rib. Ignore the cracking noises and you'll probably gain a centimetre or two. In six weeks of Pa Tuan Tsin you will have gained 60 centimetres, smooth as a swallow in flight.

If all this sounds strenuous, and if you are out of condition it no doubt is, remember that you have not just completed a course of difficult isotonic exercise. All you have done is a deep knee bend, turned your head and spread your arms properly ... all perfectly natural movements that hardly call for therapeutic instruction or medical supervision.

As we were saying, these little twinges of concern or even guilt that arise when we realise we are not giving our bodies a reasonable chance of carrying us through a long and lively lifetime, pass as quickly as they crop up. Lethargy, refusal to face the facts or just being too busy to do anything about it are the reactions that usually smother sudden bouts of determination. Another junk lunch, another drink and another smoke will make it go away. It's so much easier to convince yourself that you don't really feel that bad. In fact, most of the time, you feel pretty damn good, except when you put yourself to a simple test or two.

In my case that climb to the hilltop, with all its palpitations, was the crunch. It didn't pass. Not this time. I knew it never would unless I did something about it. I'd finally been hit by that bus and unless I got up, it was going to run right over me and back again. Then, as is so often the case in important stages of life, fate, destiny, God or just plain luck, took a hand. I met a man who impressed me with his being, changed my attitudes towards life and health with his example and pointed me in the right direction.

THERE IS NO SUCCESS WITHOUT HEALTH

Disease, dullness, indecision, carelessness, sloth, worldliness, mistaken views, losing the way and instability — these splurgings of the mind are obstacles and coexist with disordered inbreathing and outbreathing.

Patanjali

PART TWO

ENTER MR WU

I was at a meeting the day after the blowout on the Batangas road. Some smart young account director was on his well-shod feet, flashing cufflinks and research findings at a row of grim-faced money-men. I wasn't listening.

Later, after the meeting and at the sumptuous hotel lunch I'd become so accustomed to, my health and lifestyle was still on my mind. My health was on the way out and with it, my confidence. It was over the coffee and cognac that I decided to do something about it. I refused a cigar and a refill. It was a start. I had already bought my tracksuit and running shoes when into my life came Mr Wu. It is important that you share my first impressions of him and the way our relationship developed and why.

He had not attended the morning's session or the sumptuous luncheon. Mr Wu was a new addition to the agency's list of impressive clients. The securing of his business, in which I had played a major hand, caused great excitement. He was known simply as Mr Wu and his executives, the usual shifty, insecure bunch of yes-men, spoke of him in whispers, either through reverence or fear.

He arrived at the afternoon meeting, punctually. As the company rose like the fourth form greeting their headmaster, he moved swiftly to his chair at the head of the table, issued a brief but pleasant smile and a nod and sat down. Dispensing with the usual insincere handshakes and meaningless introductions, he poured himself a glass of water and by his very bearing indicated that the presentation should begin.

I had been flown across the world to show this man how to make more money, and to prepare my recommendations I had been given access to the archives of his company. It was not the usual assignment. His company had an unusual history, and Mr Wu was a most unusual man. He was extremely rich: beyond speculation, it was said. He was a Fukien Chinese who had started life as the son of a penniless woodsman in the hills of Shantung on mainland China. It was there, the story went, that he discovered the secret of ginseng ('the elixir of life') and other powerful and mysterious herbs and preparations that to the Western world represent Chinese medicine.

Now he owned a chain of stores throughout Southeast Asia, his warehouses supplied exclusively from Red China. From this had grown, among other businesses, one of the largest and most successful export companies in Asia, the Sun Moon Export Company. It was this vast enterprise that he now wished to develop and diversify into European and American markets. It was my job to advise him.

In the delicate business of bringing together buyer and seller from two totally different worlds, it has always been one of my opening tactics to make a thorough study of the personality I am being paid to impress and convince. This had not been possible with Mr Wu. I had been carefully, almost fearfully briefed by his top executive. The president, it appeared, was still far more enamoured with the earthier aspects of his herbal empire than the dalliances of the board room. His business had grown through knowledge of his product, the Chinese brilliance in business and not a little luck, timing, risk and confidence in himself and his destiny. He was far more likely, I was told, to be found chatting and taking tea in a backstreet Chinatown store or off on a field trip to Canton, than enthroned in an air-conditioned office or conference room.

I watched him closely during preliminary niceties, which he suffered in polite discomfort. He was a quiet man, with the neat, medium build of most northern Chinese, and appeared particularly well-knit and lithe under the sombre, perfectly-tailored business suit. He scarcely spoke and was hard put to conceal impatience, but he radiated an awe-inspiring sense of power. The aura of sheer energy seemed to surround him like a force. Not one of his subordinates spoke unless he addressed them with a glance or a question. Their eyes, slippery with caution, seldom left his face. No one smoked, a blessing in that badly-ventilated tomb of a room, with its mock leather chairs, projection screen and ancient air-conditioners bumbling along like muted bus engines. Mr Wu did not approve of smoking. He had requested that no one smoke and that only water or Chinese tea be served instead of the usual overdose of instant coffee and fancy biscuits.

He listened with growing intolerance to the stammered strategies and rehearsed recommendations on how he should spend a million dollars on the infiltration of foreign markets. If he was impressed or disgusted, pleased or disappointed, it was impossible to say. Only by the slight movement of his head, the sudden, piercing challenge of his eye and a rare change of expression could his understanding or approval be gauged.

He was by no means a domineering man. On the contrary, his presence had a strangely calming effect upon what usually becomes a clamorous conflict for self-justification and puerile pettiness. He seemed to fill dynamically his place at the head of the table, almost appearing to oscillate power-waves at will. His English was measured and nearly perfect; his words precise and lyrical in the old Chinese way. His gaze was fixed unflinchingly upon his subject until bored. His reactions transmitted little currents up and down the polished slab of acacia that served as a board table.

I had sat at many such meetings throughout the money centres of Asia during the previous decade, many of them attended and conducted by taipans of this man's magnitude; mysterious men who maintained a wolfish control of business throughout most of the region. Never had I been as impressed or affected as I was by the presence of Mr Wu.

The campaign I had devised for the Sun Moon Export Company was simple, directly and accurately aimed at its target without frills or flounces. It was the kind of communication I felt certain Mr Wu would understand and accept. I was right. His nods were frequent and, at appropriate points in the presentation, I was rewarded with the rarity of a smile. From him, it was an accolade. Nerves were a condition I had conquered long before, yet from the opening moments, pinned by those unshifting eyes, I felt my bowels weaken at the thought of failure.

Another trick I had learned in ten years of Asian advertising was to do my homework thoroughly, to make an in-depth study of the product I was to sell and the consumer considered most likely to go out and buy it. I had spent a week closeted in my hotel room with every book I could find on Chinese medicine and herbal remedies. As it happened I had been a keen collector of Taoist poetry and I had found a place in the campaign to quote a piece that I felt symbolised the efforts of a particular tranquillising mixture. It goes like this:

> *Bamboo shadows sweep the stairs,*
> *but the dust is undisturbed.*
> *The moonlight penetrates deep into the pond,*
> *but leaves no trace in the water.*
>
> *The wind ceases, yet blossoms continue to fall.*
> *Birds sing, yet the valley becomes quieter.*
> *In the bamboo groves, my thatched house is built by rocks.*
>
> *Through openings among stems of the bamboo,*
> *the distant village is seen.*
> *I take it easy all day, and receive no visitors,*
> *but the pure breeze sweeps a path leading to my door.*

It worked. His parting words were a gift, 'For a man who is not Chinese, you have great perception.'

It was some weeks later, when the execution of the campaign had been completed, approved and scheduled that the real honour came. A stiff square envelope containing his personal notepaper and a freely scrawled invitation to visit his home during the weekend.

He was swimming when I arrived. Long casual strokes up and down the turquoise length of his pool with the leisurely grace of an otter. I was not offered alcohol but the cold juice of calamansi, the little round lime of the Philippines, and a dish of pickled quail eggs. His servants were graciously efficient in the way I imagined of old China, their black-slippered feet silent as bare soles on the sawn stone flagging of the patio.

He completed several laps while I sat in comfortable cane and admired the rare golden coconut palms that shaded the pool. A profusion of flowers invaded the high walls of his garden in the costly privacy of Makati's Millionaire Village. Bougainvillea of every colour battled for prominence and the uncut lawns were scattered thickly with the perfumed heads of frangipani. Hibiscus blooms as big as dinner dishes spread in pink, white, scarlet and deep apricot.

He hoisted himself effortlessly from the pool and accepted a towel. There had been time to see his body before he covered it. Finely balanced, hairless and smooth as a woman's, the contours of a dancer. Across the conference room, stiff and unbending in the dark suit, I had taken him to be in his well-preserved fifties. Now, moving as he did with great flexibility, his physique seemed that of a much younger man.

During the course of an intriguing afternoon I discovered two fascinating things about Mr Wu. Firstly, that he had been a keen student of the Chinese martial art of *Wu Shu* (wrongly thought of as *Kung Fu*) since his early childhood in the forests of China. And secondly, the astonishing fact that he was almost seventy years old.

'Yours was the fifth such presentation I have listened to in past weeks. Most of them made me despair. You are the first who has taken the trouble to try and understand your subject.'

I waited. It was not enough. This, after all, was my business.

'I do not believe in advertising,' he continued, 'the goods I trade in are nature's gift. They do not need to be sold like soap and cigarettes. They sell themselves. I have never before considered it but my advisers say that I must. I leave such things to them.' He sipped, pausing just long enough to do so. 'I think your work will introduce my products to the West in a manner of which I will approve. Your approach is sensitive, even artistic. It is worthy of my confidence and I thank you for it.'

It was still not enough.

'It is not the money that will be made,' he smiled. 'Not entirely. There are many health secrets that were used in China when your people lived in caves. It is time they were shared.' Again the smile. 'If they also make me richer ...' he raised his hands in submission.

'There is one thing more. Something I can do for you in return. I was trained in my profession by a great Master, my father. He taught me many mysterious things, among them the ability to read a man's inner condition through the ancient art of facial diagnosis. Yours is not good. If you wish, I will help you. But you must be patient, very patient. And you must believe in yourself.'

There the conversation had ended.

Mr Wu's acceptance of me over a considerable period and many lengthy discussions opened doors that until then had been closed to non-Chinese. I saw him many times after that first hot Manila afternoon of calamansi juice, quiet conversation and pickled quail eggs. There were quiet dinners, sometimes at his home, but usually in the private rooms of Chinatown's backstreet restaurants. He introduced me to the rigorous scaldings and scourings of the true Shanghai bath. We were attended only by males, powerful Shanghainese whose fingers took you apart piece by piece and put you back together again, ready for the road.

Our discussions were almost always a balance of tension and relaxation, humility and ego, gentleness and aggression, tolerance and impatience, turbulence and quietude, resulting in the question of defence and attack. I was his pupil more than his friend. He probed first my outer ego, my reactions to violence, my opinion of myself, my attitude to others. With patience and always politeness, he reached into places and feelings I had not considered for years. I think he dug up what remained of my soul. I was not always aware of being tested as well as instructed.

His philosophy of life, ambition and attainment was clear-cut: without absolute health, there was nothing worth having. And to him, the discovery, understanding, development and preservation of Ch'i was the keystone around which all else was built. To attain Ch'i was like building a new foundation to replace or renew support of one that had become weakened by time and its ravages. On either side of Ch'i, holding the keystone firmly in place, there must be two things: patience and discipline. Patience above all with yourself, your own body and its limitations.

Patience breeds discipline, discipline breeds fortitude, fortitude conquers uncertainty and replaces it with confidence. From this wellspring of confidence that can be tapped in every human spirit flows the river of physical and mental wellbeing. This, he assured me in all seriousness, was that which had been sought since time immemorial as the fountain of youth. He talked of holy men who reached beyond the physical to the spiritual: Indian gurus prolonging their existence into well over one hundred and sometimes two hundred years in the rarefied air of the Himalayas, mountain peasants of Russia and Mongolia, great sages of China, lamas of Tibet, Buddhist monks of Thailand and throughout Southeast Asia, bomos of Malaysia and Indonesia, Shinto priests of Japan and the ancient order of samurai. All of them sought long life in which age brought strength and power rather than weakness and decay. All were men of the East and all, he pointed out, practised and mastered the art of breath control. As if to demonstrate the fact or perhaps explain it, he gave me the following poem:

When the mind is detached, the place is quiet.
I gather chrysanthemums under the eastern hedgerow
And silently gaze at the southern mountains.
The mountain air is beautiful in the sunset.
I drink of it as from a snow-fed stream.
It purifies me, it strengthens me, it calms me.
It becomes a river within me.
Its tributaries refresh and renew sinew, bone and marrow.
It is one with my blood
In time it becomes a torrent
To be summoned up as a storm upon the mountain.
This torrent is the fuel of life.
It is called by the masters, Ch'i

Such thoughts and discussions, very briefly summarised, formed the basis of Mr Wu's philosophy. All that is to follow came from knowing him.

THE
BROTHERHOOD
氣

The address on the envelope Mr Wu gave me led to a disused office block on the Chinatown waterfront. This is the old part of Manila, known as the Escolta, in the heart of the downtown business area. Once the scene of bitter fighting between Chinese and Filipino and still entered with a certain amount of caution by non-Chinese, it is a classic Hollywood film location.

Tugboats, barges, bumboats and scows of every length, beam, tonnage and state of repair bumped about on the khaki currents of the Pasig River. It was hard to see where the river stopped and the town began. Scavengers' huts squatted on its banks in a patchwork of stolen lumber and flattened oil drums, observation posts for the streams of flotsam that swirled in the wakes of passing river craft. The squatters gave way to cars, the cars to concrete. Noodle shops, tea shops, beauty and barber shops cohabited with sheet metal workers, tinsmiths, mechanics, hardware and the daytime dungeons of the night-time bars.

I moved with the tide of people. Five Chinese to every Filipino, flooding the narrow streets in conflicting eddies and whirlpools. The ever-building, ever-adding overflow of Chinatown, a commotion of metal on metal, wood on wood, the revving of engines, the clatter of horse-drawn calasas, a whiff of old Spain in the den of the Oriental, the tumult of dialect, the stench of heat and humanity.

A blind bootblack guarded the unswept stairs I was searching for. Beside him, the buckled cage of an antique lift crouched among its intricacies of iron trellis and ungreased cables. I decided to take the stairs. Past smells of boiling noodles and frying fat, one barred and unused door after another, welded fast with grime. I mounted empty floor after empty floor.

From above, perhaps two floors up, came sounds. The soft thump of muffled footfalls striking old floorboards, advancing and retreating to a rhythmic chant, stopping and starting to barked commands. I decide to pause and gather myself. Five flights had me out of breath.

It wouldn't do to present Mr Wu's letter of introduction with unsteady hand or answer questions with a gasp and a wheeze.

I sat on the stair to consider and felt strangely alone. Suspended between those deserted, rat-ridden rafters, echoing with age, was I right to be here? I had seldom in my lifetime felt so uncertain of my surroundings, so lost and so unimportant, never so unsuited to a time or place. I could turn back and save making a fool of myself. Back to the club with its airy bar under the cooling ceiling fans. Nothing to contend with but a procession of ice-cold San Miguel beers, people frolicking in the pool and the activity of the tennis court. I could sit at the bar watching someone else put in all the effort. I almost convinced myself all this discipline and patience was all right for fanatics like Wu. He was born to it; such effort was suited to his beliefs. He was cut out for its demands, it was part of his blood, bone and marrow. Did I really want to go on?

I thought of the chaps at the club. Men like me, who ate and drank far too much and exercised too little. Most of them were expatriates or regular travellers. Life in the East was often a trap for them. There were those that couldn't leave because they did their business there and those that couldn't stay away because the place and the people they returned to were pale by comparison. There is often glamour in places where you are not really meant to be and boredom where you belong.

The sounds from above brought me back. The stair was hard. There were cobwebs in the grille in the lift well.

'It will not be necessary for me to accompany you. Master C. is an old friend. This letter is all you will need to give him. I think he will accept you on my judgment.' Mr Wu had given me the letter a week or two before, the evening before leaving on an extended trip to China. 'You must make up your own mind if you are to use it. I can only direct you to the foot of the mountain, I cannot make you climb.'

His genuine interest in my health had been something that had seemed to evolve quite naturally from our casual acquaintance. The day had come when he had shown his concern after a vigorous game of pelota, a sort of Filipino version of squash played with a short-handled racket. I was badly out of breath and had shown it. He had observed my state with a slight frown of concern.

Later, he had put me to some basic tests. Tests, he admitted mildly, that would not be recognised by Western doctors. They were, in fact, outlawed in the British colony of Hong Kong, even though they were a thousand years older than any European method of diagnosis. No, he was not a doctor, he allowed, but in his lifetime study of herbalism and practice of Wu Shu he had learned to recognise most of the things likely to go wrong with a man. He had seen irregularities in my appearance, he explained. I was not to be alarmed, the appearance of most Western men he had observed showed a lack of knowledge of their own bodies.

'There is nothing seriously wrong with you,' he had announced with satisfaction on finishing his tests, all of which had begun and ended with the lightest touching of various parts of my body. 'I have been reading your silent pulse. You have two, you know. The silent one is the one that tells everything.'

I was overweight, he said solemnly, my wind was down, joints stiff, sinews taut, muscles soft, circulation sluggish, blood pressure erratic, respiration at half speed, liver enlarged, kidneys coping inadequately, spleen and bladder weakening and extended, heart overloaded and underpowered and lungs working at half capacity. None of which was doing my nerves any good. I was, he assured me gently, a typical Western specimen of middle-aged man. He laughed aloud at my reaction.

'Of course I exaggerate, but not so much. All of those things will befall you in the next five to ten years unless they are prevented now. It is never too late.'

His decision to send me to Chin Wu had seemed a casual one. Now I realised it was not. I had been under observation for many months. 'I cannot be sure that you will be accepted. You are non-Chinese.' He laughed. 'You would be the only foreign devil in the class.'

Mr Wu had been checking the contents of his briefcase before leaving for the airport. 'I believe that what you may learn you will put to good use. I do not say they can make a boy of you, but they can make you feel like one.'

We shook hands. 'It is now up to you.' Then he was gone.

The Chinese man who took the letter from me was of medium height, weight and build, with a pleasant but expressionless face. He was too polite to show surprise at being confronted by a foreigner. He asked me to sit while he read the letter, which was unexpectedly long. Several pages in Mr Wu's neat hand. While he read, I looked around the cubicle of an office, its walls lined with photographs of martial artists in action, ancient drawings and documents, silk banners embroidered with Chinese characters. Distant street sounds filtered up through slanted open windows.

In the gym itself, I could see perhaps twenty men. Mainly Chinese, with a sprinkling of Filipinos, they were practising ballet-like movements upon the long, wide stretch of empty floorspace. They wore loose-fitting, baggy pants, the traditional black canvas Chinese slipper and the scarlet sash of Chin Wu. Sandbags and punching blocks hung from the roof beams and an intriguing array of ancient weaponry flanked the walls: tridents, lances, spears, staves, leather armour and swords of all shapes, neatly racked.

There was a surprising lack of the effort, sweat and sound usually found in a gym. Instead, the padded footfalls were accompanied by the pervading scent of sandalwood. A spray of joss sticks flowered from a brass incense burner before a shrine which guarded the entrance to the training space.

In the five minutes that followed, I watched astounding feats of sheer, unbelievable power. I saw speed and grace combined in a way I had never imagined. Leaps of 2 to 2.5 metres from a standing position. Kicks that packed the power of pile-drivers at impossible angles and heights, while others gently performed the ballet-like movements of Tai Chi.

During my years in Asia, I had followed the martial arts as a keen and envious spectator. I had watched bouts of Tae Kwon Do in Korea; Kendo, Sumo and Aikido in Japan; Karate in Hong Kong and Singapore; Arnis in the Philippines. Once, as far back as 1945, I had witnessed an old and feeble-looking man defeat all comers aboard an allied troopship: United States marines, British commandos, Australian diggers. He had invited them all to challenge him. One, two, three or even four at a time. They had tried for an hour but not one could lay a hand on him. He had picked up the stakes, bowed politely, and moved on to the next ship.

The memory of the old man had stayed with me for a quarter of a century, and now, in this barren square on top of an abandoned office block in Manila's Chinatown, I knew I was looking at the source of his power. I was observing the training methods of the authentic art of Wu Shu in one of its many forms — The Praying Mantis.

The sound of a striking match made me turn. The Chinese had crumpled the letter into a ball. He set the match to it and when it had caught, let it drop into the incense burner.

'I have read the letter from brother Wu. We will think about it. You must come back in one week.'

I passed the blind bootblack seven times in seven weeks before I was accepted by Chin Wu. At each visit, I was courteously asked the same questions, by different instructors.

Why did I wish to learn? Was it for self-defence? Was it for health alone that I sought to develop Ch'i? How did I respond to violence, to insult, to indignity and injustice? Could I stand pain? Would I conceive of killing? Yes, they knew what had been written in the letter from brother Wu. They must hear it from me and judge for themselves. They must be sure. My answers were always the same: I was interested in the health aspects only, I would defend but never attack; in order to be gentle one must be strong (quoting Mr Wu). On the eighth visit, I was admitted. I had passed the test of patience and proved my interest by returning eight times without a sign of protest.

THE OATH

It was dark by the time they were ready for me. Outside, the noise of Chinatown had changed its tone for the night. Leisure sounds and traditional Oriental music singsonged out from tea shops and restaurants. From the bars, jukeboxes peddled the latest Western hits, the clamour of the day's business had slowed down to the brightly lit bustle of evening. Neon lights, late shops, the flames from curbside stoves and over the river shadows with an occasional glimpse of lamps and pitch flares lit up the night. The last of the students had dressed and gone. I waited. Watching the calasas pass each other on Jones Bridge, polished brass side-lights burning tiny, orange oil flames. They mixed like sparks with the street lamps. Master C. appeared at the gym door.

'We are ready for the ceremony. If you do not feel ready, we can wait.'

I had been given a brief lecture on the background of Chin Wu and its purpose, and an oath that I was asked to memorise. It seems appropriate to repeat it here as it is an indication of the true meaning of the traditions and the attitude demanded by its followers. It is very different from the popular concept of flying foot and iron fist promoted for the theatre-going audience in the making of 'Kung Fu' movies. Brutality and violence are hardly conjured up by these centuries-old words devised in the monasteries of Shaolin:

Hear me. Having been accepted as a novice of the Chin Wu school,
I hereby give my word and pledge to abide by all its regulations and
laws, to revere its ideals, to render honour and obedience to my teachers
and to practise my art with all diligence, fortitude and patience.
I swear never to reveal the secrets of my learning to
anyone without permission.
I swear never to misuse the knowledge and the power that I will receive.
I swear to comport myself at all times with quietude and humility,
that I may, through stillness, gain the peak of the mountain.

To witness this solemn oath, I invoke my lineage upon this earth,
the generations of my ancestors. I call upon the forces that
substance and move the universe.
So that if this oath I betray, their vengeance shall be upon me.
Help me!

I was asked to write the oath on a sheet of red paper and to enter the gym with it when I had finished. The area was silent and black, lit only by the two red and gold dragon candles burning on either side of the shrine. From their light, I could see the four instructors sitting motionless and straight-backed on a bench against the wall.

The ceremony took perhaps ten minutes. I was led through it with whispered words and gestures from a senior instructor. Before the twin gods of Heaven and Earth, backed by the disciples of War and Peace, Violence and Non-violence, I was asked to kowtow. With my forehead pressed to the floor, I repeated the oath and then, at a signal, burned my oath in the brass urn below the shrine. I then lit joss and presented it to each of the Gods in turn. The instructors rose with Master C. and presented me the honour of the Shaolin bow, the outstretched right fist shielded by the curved, open palm of the left, symbolising the sun and the moon. Returning it as I had been shown, I was given the Chin Wu uniform and the card that registered me as a novice of the Chin Wu Athletic Association with its Hong Kong headquarters. I had arrived at the foot of the mountain.

In the many hundreds of times I climbed those still unswept stairs to look down from its windows upon the hustle of the docks, I learned a great deal that would be pointless and tedious to include in this book. My personal emotions along the journey back to good health are unimportant. It is enough to say I was a brother of Chin Wu and as such responsible for my own progress or lack of it. Patience, discipline and fortitude, the foundation that Mr Wu had so often mentioned, began to take on practical meaning. I will not pretend it was not difficult at first. The doubts, hopes, strivings, obstacles, misgivings and sheer lethargy that had to be overcome were exclusively my own.

THE FIRST MONTH

The first three training sessions at Chin Wu were given over to lectures on the origins of the school and the traditions of Oriental martial arts. A fascinating formula of Chinese characters, hexagrams, mystic symbols and historical dates would cover the blackboard, as the ancient sources of physical and spiritual power were carefully, if briefly, unfolded. The intangible was explained, the mysterious revealed in transcriptions and translations of documents and scrolls as old as civilisation. Great Masters were talked of and their accomplishments discussed. Protocol was considered and observed.

We were taught to respect the opinion of our instructors as absolute; their attitude towards us, we were told, would always be tolerant but firm. 'You are all brothers. There is no competition among brothers, you will compete only with yourselves. There is no room for ridicule among brothers, only ridicule of yourselves. You must be gentle but stern with each other. Above all you must be gentle but stern with yourselves.'

No session began until each student had bowed three times and lit joss to the Gods of the Shrine on entering the gym. No sessions ended without the sacred salute being given by the Master and returned by his class. No student could leave the gym without bowing to the Shrine on his way out. We were taught the significance of the salute, the balled right fist shielded by the cupped left palm and held before you. This represented the sun/moon symbol of the ultimate Ch'i, the universe from which all power is drawn, and into which all power returns. The bow, so strictly enforced on entering and leaving, was the traditional Oriental prayer posture of palms pressed together and held before the heart with bowed head. This sign of absolute humility shared by Chinese, Thai, Hindu and many other Asian cultures, indicates 'respect for the light that shines within you' and is given after completion of any set of exercises. It is said also to represent the mountain which resides within each of us, waiting to be climbed.

Training began on the fourth session. Students were expected to attend twice a week and three times if possible. They were also expected to practise for at least an hour daily those exercises they had been taught and to demonstrate their progress at the next session. We began with the stances and postures, exercises designed to strengthen the legs and develop balance, position the body for movement and sharpen reflexes. They were extremely hard at first, being totally foreign to any stance or position one would normally take. We were constantly encouraged by the watchful and ever-patient instructors.

'It is good to stand a little discomfort. If there is no discomfort there can be no progress.'

'The heart of a lion cannot go far on the legs of a chicken.'

I sweated miserably and it seemed to me that I suffered alone. They were all so much younger, these rubber-boned Chinese and Filipinos. Each novice endured in his own way. A wonderful feeling of comradeship quickly grew and was nurtured by the instructors. It was truly a brotherhood: one looked upon the other with interest and concern for his progress. Challenge was posed only by the will and the heart. Conflict only showed in each man's struggle with his own body and mind. It forged respect and liking that I had never experienced in any similar Western situation.

The key to it all was patience. The Chinese characters for patience and fortitude were stitched in gold on crimson banners and hung throughout the gym, so that no matter which way you faced you could not help but see them. Of the class of twenty, three students dropped out in the second week, two in the third and another in the fourth. Master C. only smiled. 'It is always the first month that is critical. Those that are still here after the fourth week will be with us on the twenty-fourth week.'

When the stances and postures had been thoroughly taught and practised at home or outdoors, they were tested for stability and we moved on to the sequence of warm-up exercises that are a prelude to every training session. With the stances 'beginning to take root', the warm-up exercises were not as difficult to achieve. Stiff joints, sinews and muscles, slack or taut through lack of proper use soon began to tone up with simple attention to neck and shoulders, arms, hands, waist and back, legs and feet. Each exercise was repeated sixteen times, counting under the one breath, one, two, three, four, five, six, seven, eight; eight, seven, six, five, four, three, two, one.

With the stances, postures and warm-up exercises well established by the fourth week of training, the class was considered ready to begin learning *Pa Tuan Tsin — The Eight Precious Sets of Exercises*. The history of these ancient breathing exercises was presented to us by Master C. with a sincere reverence which immediately set them apart from ordinary physical endeavour. The essence of Pa Tuan Tsin, he impressed upon us, was spiritual, and although its source was a gentle and a lucid one, its summit was the crystallised power of Ch'i.

He rationalised this with an ancient Chinese credo which, roughly translated, went like this:

In order to be gentle
one must be strong.
That is why each arm must be a spear.
In order to be strong
one must be prepared.
That is why each hand must be an axe.
In order to be prepared
one must be confident
This is why every finger must be a dagger.

Many such axioms were used to demonstrate the health properties of these exercises and how they related to the violent aspects of the martial arts. They were, after all, no matter how humane their original purpose, the springboard for the most lethal and physically demanding procedure ever devised.

The breathing exercises and the harmonious body movements that accompany them were taught slowly and methodically by Master C. They were checked continually by the instructors who measured the rise and fall of a diaphragm with the back of a hand. The main problem, which seemed to be shared throughout the class of beginners, was shortness of breath. No one seemed to have the lung capacity to accommodate the prolonged inhalation and exhalation essential to concentrated breathing.

'Never mind,' said Master C. encouragingly, 'After one month of practice each morning, your breath will be like the breeze through a pine wood and your step will be light as a child's.'

He was right.

I tell you this because, to a lesser degree, you will find the first few sessions similarly difficult. I say to a lesser degree because you will be your own taskmaster, less exacting and demanding of yourself than Master C. or the instructors of Chin Wu would be. You will have no one to answer to but yourself, no instructor to face but the pages of this book, no guilt or disappointment in your efforts and progress but your own, no one to cheat but yourself. But that first critical month will be as much your testing period as if you are attending classes under their all-seeing eyes. It is from this self-control, self-appraisal and solitary judgment that discipline, willpower and certain success come with the practice of Pa Tuan Tsin. But first, there are certain basic things to be considered.

FACTS AND FANTASIES

It is important to explain further why the images created by the Western concept of Kung Fu and those demanded by the words of the traditional oath are so tremendously different. There must be no confusion between the content and purpose of this book and the combat aspects of the widely publicised martial art shown on television, in movies and in scores of books and magazines.

Kung Fu (or the Cantonese pronunciation 'gung fu') simply means 'close application ... to excel'. It signifies dedication and skill in a particular field. One can, to the Chinese mind, possess Kung Fu in cooking, sewing, sculpting or painting in exactly the same way as it is nowadays so spectacularly applied to the ancient art of Chinese Temple Boxing.

Kung Fu first became known to Americans in the early sixties, when a Chinese practitioner living in the United States published a series of books on the subject. His name was James Lee and his company, Oriental Book Sales, was the first not only to print books in English on the art of Chinese Temple Boxing, but also to reveal the technique and detail of its secrets to the Western world. He called it Gung Fu. About this time, the little-known Bruce Lee arrived from Hong Kong. Already a master of several forms of martial arts, the amazing Bruce Lee soon became a popular figure among the Karate circles of America. Until that time Karate and the Japanese forms of Ju Jitsu and Judo were all that was generally known of Oriental fighting styles.

Incredible tales of Chinese hand-to-hand fighting had been filtering into the American karate community from returned GIs who had witnessed it in the war theatres of Korea and Vietnam. It was said that against it even the lethal Tae Kwon Do of the Koreans was no match.

Bruce and James Lee decided to team up and, with James's publishing contacts plus the tenacity and talent of Bruce, they soon became the accepted authorities on all martial arts, which they called Kung Fu.

Violent film epics, such as *Big Boss, Return of the Dragon, Fist of Fury, Shaolin Avengers* and many others were soon demonstrating forbidden fighting techniques not only throughout the United States but upon every cinema screen in Southeast Asia.

Bruce Lee became the undisputed high priest of Kung Fu and the secrets of the Shaolin Temple, after eight centuries of carefully guarded silence, became available to the West for the price of a ticket.

Kung Fu 'clubs' sprang up throughout the Orient and from coast to coast across America. Very few of these followed the authentic traditions of ancient Masters. Many short cuts were taken to learn forms: techniques such as White Crane, Tiger Crane and Praying Mantis, Go Cho, Wing Chun, Tai Ch'i Chuan and Pa Kau.

The result was that without the fabled patience and discipline demanded by the old Masters, Kung Fu, after its initial but quite long-lasting dazzle, had begun to fade as all fads do. Eventually, it fell into disrepute in the eyes of Western audiences as just another phase of Oriental violence and viciousness. The popular television series starring David Carradine at least made some attempt to associate Kung Fu with the all-but-holy order taught by monks for the improvement of the physical self and betterment of the human soul.

It is so very important, when contemplating the practice of Pa Tuan Tsin, that this violent aspect be totally removed, that it is necessary to look briefly at the origin of Kung Fu.

There has always been a great difference of opinion throughout the world of martial arts as to which of the many techniques came first. What really was the original hand-fighting method that became known to the West as unarmed combat? Was it Karate, Judo, Ju Jitsu, Aikido, Kendo, Sumo, Indonesian Penjak, Thai boxing, French Savate, Korean Tae Kwon Do or Filipino methods such as Kuntao, Chako and Arnis?

The fact is that all of them sprang from the gentle art of Chinese Temple Boxing, or Wu Shu. For instance, Judo was brought to Japan by a Chinese man named Chen Yuen Too during the Ming dynasty in 1558. He taught at the Asabu Shokokuji and has a monument at the Shokoku Temple near the Japanese Imperial Palace in Tokyo. Karate came to Japan from China through Okinawa and Korea and during the Ming dynasty many Japanese studied directly under Chinese Masters.

The best way to settle this long-standing dispute is to trace the course of Kung Fu's long history through the years to its original source, Wu Shu.

SECRETS OF SHAOLIN

Take the understanding of the East and the knowledge of the West — and then seek.

Gurdjieff

PART THREE

THE MANY MOONS OF WU SHU

During the long and colourful history of China, many names and purposes have been ascribed to Chinese Temple Boxing and its numerous preliminary exercises. This history is worth tracing since it shows much of China's evolution since the first dynasty in 2200 BC. From legendary beginnings through feudal systems, wars and Cultural Revolution, the part that the original Temple Boxer played is worthy of note. Firstly, he was a mystic teacher of health preservation and spiritual arts, later an invincible warrior sought after by warlord and government alike. It was considered that one unarmed Boxer fully trained in the ways of Shaolin was worth twenty armed soldiers, and a recognised Master turned mercenary could ask his weight in gold from any general.

In earliest recorded Chinese history, this art was given recognition in the *She Ching* (Book of Poetry) as Chuan Yung, meaning 'Brave Fist'. During the Chung Chiu (Spring and Autumn Era), it became known as Wu-I (Martial Arts). The period of Chan Kuo (Warring State) considered it Ch'i (Techniques of Fighting); the Han dynasty changed it first to Ch'i Chiao (Techniques of Ingenuity) and later to Shou Po (Hand Fighting).

The Han gave way to the Wei dynasty and it became King Shou (Empty Hand). It is thought that this name and period was the beginning of Karate, which was originally known as Kung Shou Tao. With the Ming dynasty came yet other names, firstly Ch'i Yung (Techniques of Bravery), then Chi-I (Art of Techniques). The advent of the Ching dynasty brought with it the name Pai Shou (Plain Hands). The Sung dynasty (960–1279 AD) has remained famous for its art, literature and philosophy. During this highly sophisticated period original health-nourishing exercises were revived and developed as Hsing I (Internal Style of Wu Shu).

With the formation of the Chinese Republic and the gradual phasing out of ancient texts, character and cultural traditions, came Wu Shu (Martial Arts or Art of Combat), to become more widely known as Kuo Shu (National Art) and Kuo Ch'i (National Techniques). Of all these variations, Kuo Shu was generally accepted and used nationwide as a means of self-defence against foreign invasion. However, since the People's Republic of China's renewed overtures towards its Asian neighbours and the Western world, the Chinese have, for reasons best known to themselves, returned to Wu Shu, where it appears things may rest. As recently as 1977, Peking sent a delegation on a worldwide tour to illustrate the importance the Chinese place on good health through the cultural heritage of Wu Shu.

In further reference to the ancient art of Chinese Temple Boxing then, and so as to once and for all disassociate the pursuit of health and strength through Ch'i from the fighting form of Kung Fu, we too shall use the name Wu Shu for the remainder of this book.

To attempt to trace the true beginnings of Wu Shu one must remember that such information may not be accurate. The doctrine of Chairman Mao had wiped the slate clean of creed and custom, myth and legend, which had been so much a part of the Chinese spirit for centuries. Not much was left from the great book-burning to offer conclusive proof of any aspect of Chinese history. Records that did leave China were discredited and scholars were disowned. This was particularly so when it came to folklore or anything as shrouded and ancient as the source of the martial arts.

There is another reason, the Chinese say, for the lack of written evidence or literature on the subject of these arts. Since its earliest known beginnings, Wu Shu and its many diversifications were mainly developed and perpetuated by the illiterate or semiliterate classes, and therefore the information was largely disseminated by word of mouth.

A Master, or Sifu, was more likely to be found among peasant or coolie stock than among the wealthy or noble. The greatest Masters of all invariably emerged from the poor and hardy, the supposedly defenceless, particularly during the militant dynasties and the reigns of the marauding warlords of Imperial China.

The old Masters maintained that prehistoric humans, forced through lack of weaponry to hunt, kill and exist in a predatory world with nothing but bare hands and feet, were probably the very first martial artists. They were obliged to use intelligence and strength as their only means of survival. Perhaps it was then that Chuan Yuan, the Brave Fist, was first raised in defence or deadly combat.

It is accepted by most military historians that no race on earth developed and perfected the art of hand-to-hand combat more effectively than the Chinese. In their 5000 years of invasions, civil wars and revolutions, the varied inventions of weaponry and fighting techniques were perfected and practised. Although these combat skills were no doubt introduced in the interests of self-defence, the warlord eras split province from province and separated soldier from civilian more completely than anywhere else in the world.

As far back as 400 BC, the Chinese peasant saw the growing need for unarmed defence against the well-equipped, well-trained soldiers who were never far away. Some say it is here that the first forms of hand fighting were introduced and recognised. They evolved into three separate systems with completely different goals: the art of health nourishment — the development of breath control combined with sinew stretching and muscular exercise for the improvement and prolonging of life; wrestling and hand-to-hand fighting — for the purpose of self-defence; and weapon fighting — the use of club, staff, knife, axe, sword, spear, lance, trident, bow and arrow for attack and aggression.

As to the origin of the exercises you are about to learn, they are believed to have first come from India. The story goes like this: in the 1st century AD, an Indian monk arrived at the Imperial Court of China to ask permission of Emperor Leung Wu Ti to teach Buddhism in China. It was granted and he made his way to Shung San (Mount Shung) and the Shaolin monastery. He is said to have meditated before its walls for nine years before teaching what he called 'The Eighteen Hands of Lo Han', 'The Marrow-washing Course' and 'The Sinew-changing Course'. These were strictly health and inner energy methods taught to the celibate novice monks as part of their Buddhist training.

Romantic legend insists that Bodhidharma, known to the Chinese as 'Tamo' and to his disciples as 'Eyes of Eternal Summer', was also responsible for the introduction of the formidable Shaolin fighting forms. But documented scrolls prove that the first 'long hand fighting style' was attributed to a Master named Kwok Yee in the last Han dynasty (250–220 BC). So, it is unlikely that Tamo was the originator of Wu Shu or Pa Tuan Tsin.

After Tamo's death, at the age of seventy-six, the Shaolin monks he had trained continued to practise and improve on his 'Health Nourishing Exercises', in the pursuit of peace brought about by perfect health achieved through the harmony of meditation and breath control. However, like so many things developed purely for good, it was not long before it was corrupted and turned against itself.

Growing harassment by bandits and renegade warlords caused the monks to channel their incredible powers into defensive combat techniques. By the end of the bloody Tang dynasty, their amazing skills and feats of courage and strength were talked about with awe throughout China. The tranquil monks of Shaolin had become the most feared warriors on any battlefield.

As their fame spread, word of their legendary encounters became associated with mysticism and the supernatural. Not surprising when you consider the superstition that surrounds all Chinese belief and the truly 'superhuman' exploits of the defenders of Shaolin. It did not take long for the rot to set in.

During the Ching uprising of 1912, after the fall of the Ming dynasty, patriots and guerilla bands shaved their heads and retreated to the sanctuary of the Shaolin monastery. There they secretly trained in the techniques of Wu Shu until the time was right to strike back at the savage ching government.

A traitor among them betrayed the plot to the Ching administration, which sent its armies upon the loyalists in a surprise attack. In the battle that took place, the sacred Shaolin monastery was razed to the ground. For the few Masters who survived the attack, treachery and defeat served as a bitter lesson. They swore the secrets of Shaolin would never again fall into the wrong hands.

From that time, the strictest possible secrecy has been maintained. No student, no matter what his credentials, his social status or his fortune, would be accepted without absolute proof of his character and morality. This utmost caution was further protected by the severity of the oath* each novice was forced to take before being accepted into the Brotherhood. This close secrecy was enforced by the threat of death and damnation and was strengthened even more during the Boxer Rebellion of 1899.

When the eight combined imperial armies invaded China and ousted the Ching government, foreign occupation proved little better or perhaps worse than the oppression it had replaced. Enslavement and abuse of the Chinese spawned a lasting hatred for the Foreign Devil, who had 'freed them from the claws of the Ching dragon only to be devoured by the Imperialist lion'.

That hostility led to a total rejection of any contact with foreigners and all things foreign; and recognition of, or respect for, foreign customs, traditions or religions was taboo. It is not surprising that China's most precious and enduring possession, the new, diverse and highly effective variations of Wu Shu, was kept from foreign powers at all costs. The secret was, until recently, as jealously guarded as Western progress in the arms race and the conquest of space.

For the most part, this contempt and indifference still exists. It most definitely restricted traditional Chinese Masters from considering foreign students and does so to this day.

* The oath on page 32, still in use in authentic Kung Fu circles, has probably changed a little in time, but its meaning is regarded just as seriously.

Only when superhero Bruce Lee, the young, Westernised wizard of martial arts, exposed all he knew in his screen spectaculars and began teaching American enthusiasts was the long-lasting taboo broken. Even so, at the very peak of his phenomenal and unchallenged success, he is said to have been asked to stop demonstrating his mastery to the outside world. No doubt he was reminded of his oath. The mystery that surrounds his death may have come as no surprise in certain traditional Wu Shu circles.

That, very briefly, is the story of Wu Shu as it is accepted by Chin Wu and other schools of equal repute. As with all attempts to define historical events in the China of old, this version stands to be contradicted. It is, however, an attempt to give as authentic an explanation as possible, based on the evidence and opinions of those who have devoted a lifetime to the preservation and continuation of a traditional art.

To return again to the exercises contained in this book. With the death of Bodhidharma and the several centuries of unrest that followed the corruption of Shaolin, a famous soldier hero of the Sung dynasty emerged. General Yeh Fei was, as well as a brilliant strategist, a great Master of Wu Shu and reputed founder of Hsing I (Internal Style of Wu Shu). It was he who revived Tamo's Health Nourishing Exercises and developed them. It was the great physician, Hua T'o, however, who devised Pa Tuan Chin which, loosely translated, means: 'Pa' (eight), 'Tuan' (chapter), 'Chin' (different movements in a set). Chin also means 'a very precious multicoloured quilted silk'. 'Pa Tuan Chin', therefore, means 'Eight Precious Sets of Exercises', or (roughly) 'Eight Precious Sets of Silk-weaving Exercises'.

General Yeh Fei was a northerner and consequently Pa Tuan Chin became known as the Northern Style. It was considered extremely difficult to master. A less demanding Sifu from the south, known as Liao She Chiang, further refined the art of General Yeh, simplifying the movements with the same objective in mind: 'that of livening up the internal organs and arresting unhealthy symptoms in the human body'. Liao She Chiang's version became accepted as Pa Tuan Tsin, or Southern Style, and it is these exercises, unchanged for eight hundred years, that you are about to learn.

Whoever practises Pa Tuan Tsin correctly will gain the pliability of a child, the health of a lumberjack and the peace of mind of a sage.

Liao She Chiang

GREAT MASTERS OF CH'I

Although this book deals with one set of warm-up and breathing exercises often adopted in certain authentic forms of Wu Shu, it in no way claims to be an introduction to the combat/defence aspects of the cultivation of Ch'i. If only for the sheer fascination of the subject, however, it would be a pity not to touch on the lives of one or two Masters and to give examples of the all-but-superhuman powers attributed to devotees of Ch'i.

Among the many schools and countless forms of Wu Shu practised throughout China and the Eastern world, many are becoming increasingly accessible to the West. Probably because of this diversification after years of secrecy, modified techniques and improvised styles are continually appearing. Some are created for expediency and to facilitate those impatient with their progress. Others are the legitimate advancement of new forms evolving from the ancient classics, often a combination of the best elements from several famous schools.

The best example of such a form devised by a modern Master is Jeet Kune Do, the deadly and spectacular technique developed by the late Bruce Lee. Jeet Kune Do means 'Fist Intercepting Way', and was used to shattering advantage in all of his films. It was arrived at through many sources, the classical and cultural as well as the experimental application of his own brand of genius. Only an artist of Lee's magnitude could have achieved such an ambition. In order to achieve it, he utilised a lifetime of practice, which included mastery of most known styles and methods including Karate and Tae Kwon Do.

He then made a long and careful study of the human anatomy, researched deeply into biomechanics, examined muscle function and nerve reaction in finest detail, so as to concentrate on the upsetting of an opponent's centre of gravity. His later studies were dedicated to the development of unique rotary movements as the most economical way of using energy to the greatest effect — as in his famous sequence of three continuous round-house kicks.

Lee developed a high-velocity 'internal punch' technique which left little external evidence but set up mass vibrations in the body that could result in internal haemorrhaging. Such unorthodox breakaways were heavily criticised by conventional schools for lack of philosophical basis and for their eclecticism. Despite this criticism, Jeet Kune Do became accepted as by far the most visually expressive style of all. In films, it very soon eclipsed the highly contrived Chinese 'sword' movies that had for so long been the exclusive domain of Asian film-makers such as Run Run Shaw, himself a student of Wu Shu.

The persuasive and undoubtedly brilliant Bruce Lee soon convinced his director, Lo Wei, to do away with the picturesque weaponry and trick effects which has always been the most important part of the Eastern martial arts film and to bring things into the twentieth century by featuring the unarmed body alone. This would fully express the explosive force, control and grace that such action-packed epics called for. It is doubtful weather Bruce Lee or his director could have foreseen the personality cult that would arise from his decision.

Following the decline of Kung Fu movies came serious attempts to put things back in their proper context. The television series Kung Fu, starring David Carradine as Kwai Chang Caine, probably came closest to restating the age-old credo:

Avoid rather than check.
Check rather than force.
Force rather than injure.
Injure rather than maim.
Maim rather than kill.

This philosophy of patience was illustrated by Carradine's portrayal of an exile from the Shaolin Temple wandering through the American West, applying his temple training in a hostile environment with the humility and rigid principles of his Chinese teachers.

I once saw an excellent first-hand example of this same law of restraint which has left a lasting impression on me and set the seal upon my own code of ethics in such circumstances. It occurred in a noodle shop in Manila's Chinatown where I was enjoying a bowl of conjee, or rice broth, with one of the Chin Wu instructors. His name does not matter as he was an exceptionally shy and humble man and would probably not like to see his name in print. I shall call him 'D'. He was a tall young Chinese of the classic Wu Shu build combining the grace and symmetry of a dancer with the defined muscle of a weight-lifter.

He was a champion of the formidable White Crane form as well as being thoroughly schooled in the Praying Mantis and Tiger Crane. This was due to his total dedication to no less than three hours solid practice every day, a discipline that had been religiously maintained from his boyhood. At the time, he was in his mid-twenties and at the very peak of condition. The fine physique, incidentally, he claimed was owed largely to the constant practise of Pa Tuan Tsin, as he had never touched a weight in his life. He had recently returned from winning several honours at the International Martial Arts Competition in Taiwan. Master C. had told me this because, with characteristic modesty, D had not mentioned it.

The cafe was crowded with hefty-looking Chinese truck drivers, sheet metal workers and factory labourers, and D and I were lucky to squeeze into a seat. We had hardly taken a mouthful when a giant of a man, wearing the grime of an iron-worker from the nearby foundry, told my companion to give up his seat. I understood enough Cantonese to know that it was an order rather than a request and not a polite one at that ... something along the lines of, 'Why should a boy be seated while a man stands?' D ignored the insult, continuing to eat without acknowledging the remark.

The man laid it on a little thicker. 'Any Chinese who would be seen eating with a foreign devil is little better than a bar girl.' I looked around at the grinning horde and remembered that before the enforcement of martial law this area was noted for its rioting and violence. The man had a point. Seldom was a foreigner seen in the area, certainly not eating in a working man's cafe. To save the mayhem I knew D could cause in less than a second, I offered my seat. I was, after all, out of bounds. But the bully did not want my seat, he wanted D's, and was determined to take it. Reaching out he took D's bowl and emptied the contents into a spittoon with the comment that 'the boy would not be needing the rice because he no longer had a seat'.

It was a shameful insult, heard by the delighted crowd, which was on the intruder's side because of my presence, the man's size and D's youth. D could have redeemed himself in any one of a hundred spectacular ways, turning himself from a suspected coward into a hero with devastating ease. He did not. With polite apologies to me, his face a mask, he gave up his seat, purchased another bowl of conjee and ate it standing up. It was typical of the truly accomplished Wu Shu fighter, but I shuddered at what would have happened if the thug had laid a hand on my patient young friend. I encountered many such instances during my time with Chin Wu and it made me extremely proud to be even a very small part of such an elite group.

Of course, not all experts are as cool and considerate as the immovable D. The famous Johnny Chiuten, renowned as all-round champion of the Philippines in all forms of martial arts and technical adviser to Chin Wu, was also Manila's most notorious street fighter. This extract from a 1977 issue of *Martial Arts* magazine, written by an equally well-known fighter, gives an idea of his prowess.

The 'old' Johnny Chiuten fought as if he were a bullet with blades. He came at you smiling, fast, hands and feet whirling until you were reduced to helpless, aching confusion; angry at yourself and awed by the man who had just mastered you. In those days I once had the honour of sparring with Johnny in the company of about thirty other martial artists. There were times when he would take on all of us, one after the other or four at a time, teaching us while administering formidable demonstrations of speed and power. We were not such a bad bunch of street fighters, counting among us several national champions.

Johnny Chiuten had his first lessons in Wu Shu from his grandfather in Canton. These consisted of breathing exercises and stances. Over the years his fighting style has become refined and polished to a unique perfection. All excess movement has been discarded, leaving a clean irresistible thrust of amazing power. 'My Ch'i,' says Johnny Chiuten, 'is a very young Ch'i.'

I had the unexpected honour to be chosen as Mr Chiuten's partner for a demonstration of his art. I have seldom met such a polite and humble man ... whilst, of course, he smilingly cut me to pieces.

In spite of remarkable experts like Johnny and D, the most incredible stories come from the past. Legendary Masters whose feats are still talked about in Wu Shu circles the world over. Accomplishments of Ch'i that will prove hard to believe for the average Western reader, in spite of what you may have seen performed on the screen by miracle men like Bruce Lee and his successors. Regardless of what perhaps you have seen with your own eyes at exhibitions of popular fighting techniques, you will find it hard indeed to imagine the extremes to which the ancient Wu Shu Masters so determinedly cultivated their Ch'i.

It becomes impossible to separate fact from fiction or myth from legend. Perhaps it is enough to know that the members of Chin Wu and other highly respected schools believe such stories absolutely and repeat them in lecture studies throughout fundamental training.

One of the best known and most fascinating stories deals with the origin and evolution of the classic Wang Lang or Praying Mantis form of Wu Shu, the style that has always utilised Pa Tuan Tsin as its life force.

During the Ming dynasty there was a native of northern China named Wang Lang, a man of little means but great and genuine patriotism. From childhood he had hoped to be of service to his country but he was constantly rejected because of his tender age, mild appearance and slight frame.

Desperate to be of use in the growing unrest between the Ming government and the Ching rebels, he sought out the monks of the

Shaolin Temple and applied himself resolutely to the art of Temple Boxing. When the government faced almost certain defeat at the hands of the ching hordes, Wang Lang, now a grown man and possessing the martial secrets of Shaolin, again offered himself as a soldier, but he was not accepted. He was rejected once more when the government was finally toppled and the infamous Ching reign began.

His determination to uphold his beliefs undaunted, he returned to the temple to further his studies and join forces with the guerilla bands plotting to destroy the new regime. Their plans were discovered because of a traitor in their midst and, as I related previously, the temple was burned to the ground.

Wang Lang managed to escape with his beloved Sifu and they made their way across the Nga Mei and Kwan Lun mountains to Lo Shan in the Lo Province (now Shantung). He continued to learn from his Sifu until the old man died, leaving a senior colleague to take over responsibility for Wang's tutelage. For many more years he learned and practised daily with his new Master, but was never able to defeat him. Finally, he was given an ultimatum. The Master would leave the student to his own devices for a period of three years and on his return he expected the young man to defeat him with ease.

Left to continue his practice alone, Wang Lang was resting one day in the woods when his attention was attracted by a hissing sound. Above him on a low twig, a praying mantis and a large grasshopper were fighting to the death. He watched, fascinated, as the powerful arms and chisel blows of the wary mantis confounded the grasshopper. How artfully it attacked and retreated at exactly the right time, grasped and released, feinted and struck methodically and relentlessly, until the grasshopper lay dead.

Wang Lang was greatly intrigued by the way the mantis had employed long-distance strikes coupled with sudden bursts of lethal in-fighting to deliver its fatal blows. They were the tactics, he realised, of a master boxer. Without further thought he captured the mantis and took it back to the temple.

Every day he provoked the insect with a piece of straw, keenly noting the reactions and responses to such aggravation. Using his years of rigid training and practical experience, he soon discovered twelve principal methods of attack and defence employed so effectively by the mantis. He then combined these strategies with the finer points taken from seventeen other schools of Temple Boxing and consolidated them into one unique form, now known as the Northern-style Praying Mantis School of Chinese Temple Boxing.

Needless to say, when Wang's Sifu returned and challenged his pupil to the decisive bout, the Master was easily defeated and immediately adopted his pupil's new style as superior to his own or any other he had encountered. They continued to polish and innovate, combining the strength and power of the mantis with the agility and speed of the monkey, until the older man died and Wang was left to pass on his knowledge alone. He chose the monks of Shaolin, whose order had given him so much in his early years. The art was practised in strict seclusion within the walls of the temple until Wang Lang died and an abbot named Sheng Hsiao Tao Jen began teaching the mantis style in other parts of China.

Among Tao Jen's pupils was an enterprising man of great strength who, having acquired the skills, established a 'pui kuk', or security service. Using the mantis tactics, he became known throughout northern China as 'Li the Lightning Fist'. Many a robber band tried but none succeeded in subduing him and Li the Lightning Fist enjoyed a long life of fame and notoriety. Age forced him to pass on his skill to a national Wu Shu champion, Wang Yung Seng, whom he had easily defeated and who had begged to be taught his amazing style.

From Wang Yung Seng it was passed on to the most colourful fighter of all; a huge northerner weighing well over 136 kilograms, known far and wide as 'Giant Fan of the Iron Palm'. Fan was a master of Tieh Sha Chang — a feat practised by thrusting the palms into a tank of iron granules — and possessed an 'awesomely powerful Ch'i'.

His strength was famous throughout China in the 1870s but was always only connected with self-defence or defence of the weak and helpless. Impressed by the passive character of Fan, Sifu Wang decided to pass on all he knew to this gentle and deserving giant. After some years of constant private instruction, Fan was crossing a field when he was attacked by two bulls charging simultaneously from opposite directions. Noting the angle and speed of each and with a coolness that is hard to imagine, he prepared to defend himself. The record claims that the first bull went down, pole-axed by a single throat kick, and the second from one blow on the spine. Both were dead before they hit the ground.

Such a champion was bound to become widely known in the way that legendary gunfighters of the old West were known and pestered by glory-seekers. Fan was constantly accepting challenges and defeating opponents. Towards the turn of the century, he was invited to Siberia to take on the best Cossack fighters and Masters of the mystic martial arts of Mongolia. He beat all comers with ease. Then the Russians, with traditional style, trotted out their biggest gun, which they had, of course, kept till last. The pride of the Cossack cavalry was almost as big as Fan, far more ferocious and it was said that the combination of him and his great Siberian stallion was invincible against man or beast.

With a keen Russian sense of fair play, the horse and rider were pitted against the Chinese. Fan, it is claimed, stood his ground, summoned all his power with a perfectly timed breath and waited until his six-legged adversary was all but on top of him. Then, with a shout that echoed in the mountains a kilometre away, he killed the horse with a blow from his iron palm. The Russians capitulated and Giant Fan took the championship back to China.

It would be easy to dispute an example such as this on several grounds — even Muhammed Ali would think twice about making such a claim — and yet it is a reasonably modest one compared to many. As recently as the 1950s, jumps of 6 metres into the air and long jumps of 10 metres from a standing position were being reported from Mainland China and Taiwan.

Even allowing for the exaggeration of enthusiasm, and perhaps cutting such claims by half, they are still difficult to credit in the Western mind when compared to current Olympic records. Yet certain stories have persisted through the years and are accepted as gospel by the Wu Shu fraternity. Some of the most popular follow.

Yang Lu-Chu'an, the father of modern Tai Ch'i, who practised daily for most of his life and taught into his seventies, was said to have walked 3 kilometres through a rainstorm without getting a trace of mud on his boots. His son had demonstrated a similar buoyancy by rising to the ceiling to light a cigarette from the oil lamp 3 metres above him. Some fighters claimed to 'push' chairs and tables without touching them, even to walk up walls.

The effect such stories of levitation and hidden energy have had upon the Asian imagination is dramatically demonstrated in Eastern 'sword' movies where Kung Fu warriors try to out-jump and out-fly the clans of the samurai.

Separating myth from fact is not so difficult when you are in regular contact with the Brotherhood. When I once watched with amazement as an instructor completed a series of push-ups on one forefinger, he told me of various methods once used to develop the power of the fingers for 'small hand' fighting in such deadly techniques as the Tiger Claw, Eagle Beak and Crane Beak. Possible for only the most advanced Masters, death is caused by striking the 'silent pulse points'. Called the 'Touch of Death' and, fortunately, known only to an elite few, this power is easier to imagine when you have seen a man plunge finger through a wooden plank or rip open a leather punching bag with a single jab.

One such master of 'touching' practised with a 20 kilogram weight tied to his finger and regularly set it alight with lamp oil. I have seen an old man squash a potato in his fist and then, to demonstrate his control, spar with an opponent while holding a bird's egg in the hollow of that same lethal palm.

Examples of Ch'i concentrated in the belly area are common at practice sessions. A man may invite another to strike his stomach or solar plexus and use the power of Ch'i to contract and expand iron-hard muscles to 'bound off' his attacker, often with the result of a sprained or broken wrist or ankle. When you have seen a Wu Shu Master in his seventies run up the wall of a room, slap the ceiling three times and drop lightly as a cat at your side, it is all more easily believed. My own Master would occasionally demonstrate his Ch'i by 'pulling' a punch several centimetres from a thick plant of wood and snuffing out a candle on the opposite side with the force of its trajectory.

The examples are endless, each one seeming to outstrip the other. If those mentioned do no more than entertain and perhaps demonstrate the power attributed to Ch'i, when channelled into such force, they may also indicate its effect when developed for health alone.

Giant Fan, of whom we spoke earlier, continued to teach the Northern-style Praying Mantis throughout his lifetime, and two of his students were destined to emerge above all others and to perpetuate the famous name of Chin Wu. Their names were Lo Kuang Yu and Lin Ching Shan. The dedication of these two fighters and the brilliance of their teacher reached the notice of the Shanghai Committee of the Chin Wu Athletic Association. In 1919, a contest was arranged between the two and the committee was amazed by the perfection of their style. The winner, by 'an almost mystic' margin, was Lo Kuang Yu. He was escorted back to Shanghai where he was made the association's chief instructor.

In 1929, at the national championships held in Nanking, one of Lo's students, Ma Cheng Hsin, became the outright winner. Both he and his Sifu were hailed throughout China as the ultimate champions. Some years later, the Central Chin Wu Headquarters sent Lo on an inspection tour of its branches in the southern provinces, Hong Kong, Macau and throughout Southeast Asia. He returned to Shanghai until war broke out and again was sent to Hong Kong to take over the Chin Wu branch there and to continue to teach the mantis style, which he did until 1944. From among these pupils there emerged a handful of men who are now the foremost Masters of the mantis form. Among them is Master Chou Ch'i Ming who in turn taught the art to Master Shakespeare Chan, from whom I was fortunate enough to learn, among other things, the precious exercises of Pa Tuan Tsin.

It is due to Mr Chan's confidence and generosity that I have been allowed to publish this book. 'Teach others what you have learned, but no more than you have learned,' he said when I asked permission, 'but teach them first how to breathe.' He then quoted a hexagram from *I Ching* (trans. James Legge, ed. Raymond van Over, Bantam, New York, 1969) which, roughly translated, meant:

> *I do not go and seek the inexperienced, but he comes and seeks me.*
> *When he shows sincerity that marks the first recourse to divination,*
> *I instruct him.*

Let us look at the first step along the road to Ch'i: correct breathing.

THE GIFT OF BREATH AND HOW TO USE IT

I eat the air promise-crammed.
William Shakespeare

PART
FOUR

THE MEANING OF CH'I

To the average person, respiration is the effortless, automatic process of breathing in and breathing out, neither helped, nor hindered by further knowledge or confusion. You breathe in fresh air and breath out 'stale' air. It is what your biology teacher called oxygen inhalation (or inspiration) and carbon dioxide exhalation (or expiration).

Not many of us know or care much more than that. We take it for granted that this, along with other vital functions of the body, keeps us alive without our even being conscious of it. For the purpose of the exercises to come, however, it is enough to establish a few simple facts, with apologies to those who already know them.

There's a lot more to your lungs than two bags going up and down, day and night. For instance, the right one has three separate compartments, the left one two. The lower lobe, which you could say is the very bottom of the barrel, hardly gets used at all in normal shallow breathing. It should be regularly accessed, emptied of stagnant air and refilled afresh.

Each lung is infiltrated by the bronchus (bronchial tubes), leading from the trachea (windpipe) rather like branches spreading from the trunk of a delicate tree. From the branches, sprout the twigs (bronchioles) and at the end of the twigs grow the air sacs, made up of clusters of pouches (alveoli), rather like bunches of grapes. Oxygen is channelled via an intricate network of air canals from the larynx to the alveoli. If that oxygen supply route were to be cut off like sap on a vine, the grapes would wither and die. Add to this the scores of vital elements that make up and maintain the entire respiratory system and there's more to breathing than meets the nostrils.

We may not know it, but we breathe in two distinctly different ways for two totally different purposes, both at the same time. Air does not just enter and leave the lungs (known as external respiration), it also distributes oxygen throughout the body via the bloodstream, unlocking the doors of energy cells; this is known as internal respiration, or tissue breathing.

The simplest explanation I can give is this. We know our main source of energy comes from the sun. It is absorbed, trapped and banked for our benefit in all green plants by the process of photosynthesis. Much of the food we eat begins as green plant life: grains, cereals, fruit and vegetables. No matter how hard we may try to refine, process, boil and bother the life out of it, we end up with enough left to keep us going. This is excellent reason for increasing our intake of fresh greens, raw vegetables and fruit.

We also know that our bodies are made up of countless cells. What we may not know is that each cell stores a number of tiny 'powerhouses' called mitochondria, which have only become visible with the development of the world's most advanced electron microscopes. The rod-shaped mitochondria contain enzymes necessary to break down sugar and store it until it is needed. Oxygen is transported into the bloodstream via the capillary network. This is the internal respiration, which acts as a trigger mechanism, detonating minuscule explosions of sheer, exhilarating life force.

It is easy to see how and why our general health and physical wellbeing are directly linked to our capacity to breathe properly and to let the mitochondria do their work. This ability to control the process of breathing, to distribute oxygen to all parts of the body, to concentrate and release this power supply at will, is what the Chinese Masters call Ch'i.

It is a word that is often misunderstood, even among modern-day Kung Fu practitioners; it remains a mystery to some. To most, Ch'i is simply a three-letter word meaning physical power and is associated with health improvement and body conditioning. To them, the magic of Ch'i, with its legendary, almost occult, background, needs no further explanation or investigation.

The reason for this is simple. As with most of the martial arts, particularly the 'hard style', visually dynamic Karate, so-called Kung Fu clubs sprouted like mushrooms in the wake of Bruce Lee's fame. Often, these clubs were profit-making organisations offering crash courses in chosen techniques. They were not always under the supervision of fully qualified instructors and seldom, in the case of Kung Fu, led by a recognised traditional Master.

A club that promises a black belt in a year or two, or mastery of a Kung Fu form in record time for a set package fee, obviously proves more attractive to the impatient student than the ten or more disciplined years of authentic instruction. In such circumstances, the time involved for fundamental training and conditioning is often skipped over, sometimes left out altogether or modified in the interests of getting on with the glamorous business of shattering tiles or performing flying kicks. Too often the main purpose is violence, whether 'defensive' or not.

The few schools lucky enough to be under the supervision of a recognised Sifu attracted only those with the patience and genuine interest in the art as a culture rather than a street-fighting technique. These chosen few were fortunate enough to be taught the essential basics of Pa Tuan Tsin in the true pursuit of Ch'i. Even the little which has been intelligently written and preserved from Chinese history fails to define the true meaning of the word.

Ch'i is usually referred to as 'intrinsic energy'. But what is intrinsic energy? Most dictionaries describe the word 'intrinsic' as 'belonging naturally, inherent, essential'; and the word 'energy' as 'force, vigour, individual powers in exercise, dynamic ability'. A reasonable interpretation, then, would be: *A natural and essential power or force inherent within the individual and motivated by dynamic exercise.*

Probably the simplest and most accurate description of Ch'i is air pressure. Every movement or inner function of the human body,

THE MANDALA: THE GOLDEN FLOWER.

Believed to be the most resplendent of all flowers, it is often used in Taoist philosophy to represent the flower of life through breath.

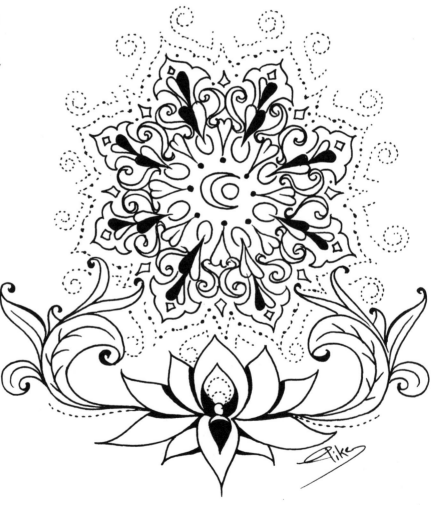

voluntary or involuntary, is brought about by manipulation of the muscles, which is impossible without internal air pressure. Bodily motion, no matter how insignificant, would cease without it. Active circulation of fresh blood, utterly essential to healthy tissue, is stimulated and regulated by this inner air pressure (tissue breathing) or degenerated and weakened by the lack of it.

Modern-day exercises have their individual benefits and offer various advantages in the increasing drive to 'keep in trim', shed excess body weight or build it up, gain energy, reduce tension, improve digestion, relieve constipation, lower blood pressure. The targets are endless and impossible to achieve through any one sport or single physical training method ... except through the development of Ch'i.

Regulated breathing or breath-control is the basic aim of any athlete, whether swimmer, runner or weight-lifter. Any endeavour that calls for excessive bursts of energy or the storing and expanding of reserve power under extreme physical effort has as its most important requirement controlled breathing.

The difference between concentrated breathing and other exercises is in the method rather than the aim. Top physical conditioning, robust health and long life are the dream of any intelligent human being. Ch'i makes this possible without the tedium of self-inflicted over-action.

The diagram on page 58 shows an unexaggerated example of the three breathing patterns: 1. shallow, or top, breathing; 2. middle breathing; 3. deep, or complete, breathing. The majority of people believe that they are breathing properly when they are inhaling and exhaling in the shallow manner illustrated in part 1 of the diagram. Many of us are quite satisfied so long as we seem to be getting enough oxygen to keep us going. On finding that we puff and gasp for air when forced to run, climb stairs or involve ourselves in sudden physical effort, we say we are 'out of breath' or 'winded'. Our respiratory system struggles to take in the unaccustomed amount of air needed to perform the exercise.

In shallow breathing, only the top compartment (one-third) of the lung is used for fresh intake of air, the other two-thirds are left to stew in the stale air from your last exertion, and perhaps the smoke from countless cigarettes. It is significant to note that tobacco smoke is always inhaled through the mouth, the cigarette, pipe or cigar acting as the filter instead of the membranes of the nostrils. Most smokers inhale very deeply when they 'draw back' the smoke, but few expel it all before the next inhalation. It is not hard to imagine what effect this has on the intricate and delicate network of the lower lung; especially overnight, when a smoker usually mouth-breathes (snores) until morning. The part of the body upon which all else relies for energy has been left to stagnate, as the early morning cough and

BREATHING
DIAGRAM
*1. Shallow breathing:
Only one-third of the
lungs being used.*
*2. Middle breathing: Two-
thirds of the lungs being
used.*
*3. Complete breathing:
Total lung capacity being
used.*

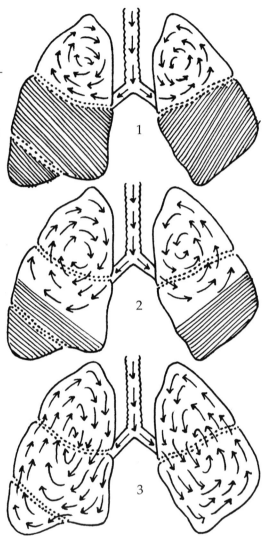

foul breath will testify. It is alarming to imagine what happens to these vital organs over a period of years, and not at all surprising that smoking is connected with malignant lung disease.

Middle breathing, or perhaps we should call it 'ordinary' breathing, uses half or two-thirds of the lung capacity but still leaves the lower compartment untouched, especially the extra lobe of the left lung which hardly ever gets cleaned out and refilled at all (this area is often the beginning of trouble). At least middle breathing makes for a better balance of oxygen, supplies more energy and helps purify the blood. It is usually the physical worker, forced to take in enough air to cope with his/her task, or the normal exerciser, who unconsciously practises middle breathing.

Deep or complete breathing is obviously the way we were meant to breathe. If not, our lungs would only be the size of the unshaded areas in the diagram. But they are not. They are there to be completely and continually filled with fresh air and emptied. 'Not practical,' you may say. 'How can I sit at my desk doing deep breathing all day?' And, of course, you'd be right. We cannot consciously practise the complete breath throughout our daily routine, and deep breathing is a conscious effort, until it becomes second nature.

No doubt in the days when people spent their time pounding across open country in pursuit of the sabre-toothed tiger, and then dragging it back to the cave after a fight to the death, heavy breathing was an automatic function. But if we cannot take off across the plains in search of action, we can at least go through the preparation before we begin our day. Even the greatest of all disciples of vital breath, the Indian yogi, realises this and begins each day with selected breathing rituals such as the 'cleansing breath'. This simply consists of raising

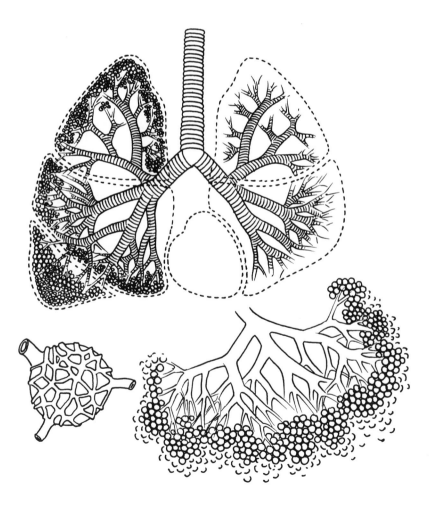

LUNG DIAGRAM
Air travels from the nose through the windpipe, or trachea, into the bronchial tubes, which divide like the branches of a tree to form the bronchioles and alveoli, the tiny air sacs which distribute oxygen into the bloodstream via the capillary network.
It is from here that the trapping and circulation begins.

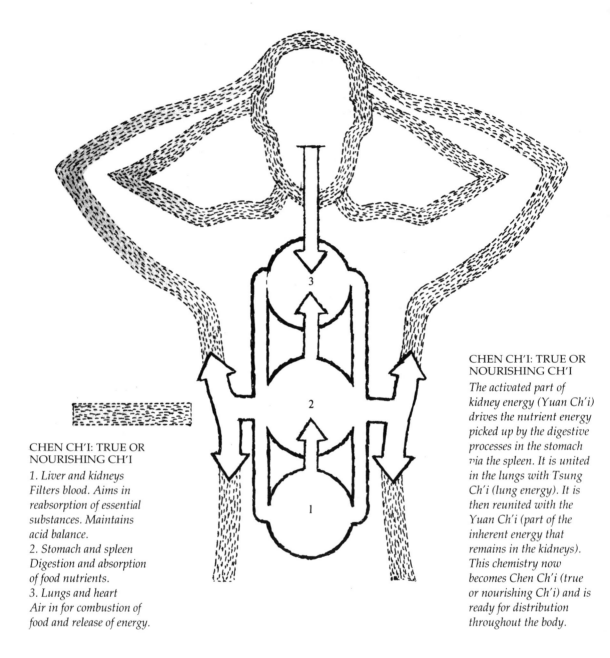

CHEN CH'I: TRUE OR NOURISHING CH'I

The activated part of kidney energy (Yuan Ch'i) drives the nutrient energy picked up by the digestive processes in the stomach via the spleen. It is united in the lungs with Tsung Ch'i (lung energy). It is then reunited with the Yuan Ch'i (part of the inherent energy that remains in the kidneys). This chemistry now becomes Chen Ch'i (true or nourishing Ch'i) and is ready for distribution throughout the body.

CHEN CH'I: TRUE OR NOURISHING CH'I

1. Liver and kidneys
Filters blood. Aims in reabsorption of essential substances. Maintains acid balance.
2. Stomach and spleen
Digestion and absorption of food nutrients.
3. Lungs and heart
Air in for combustion of food and release of energy.

the clasped hands above the head while inhaling deeply and then throwing the upper body violently forwards and downwards to expel any stale air gathered overnight. Sometimes called the 'wood chopping' exercise because the movement suggests chopping a log, the cleansing breath is repeated a half dozen times at the start of yoga classes.

Only when we have learned to fill and empty our lungs in the way nature intended, can we begin to develop the inner, or tissue, breathing that leads to the cultivation of Ch'i.

Known originally as 'Chi Kung', the art of cultivating air pressure within the body, Ch'i is the practice of certain breathing techniques, beginning in the mind and eventually transported to the body's centre of specific gravity, the lower abdomen. This is a point 5 to 8 centimetres below the navel, which the Chinese call 'tan tien'. The person who accomplishes this technique preserves health, sustains youth and is able to call upon extraordinary reserves of inner strength. He/she can summon up split-second reflex action and explosive power, incomprehensible to the average human being.

Such a state is only reached by years of arduous and dedicated training and it would be foolish to pretend otherwise. There are many stages and variations in the climb to the ultimate Ch'i and there are no grades, distinctions or belts to encourage progress, only your own improving health and increasing confidence. Pa Tuan Tsin improves

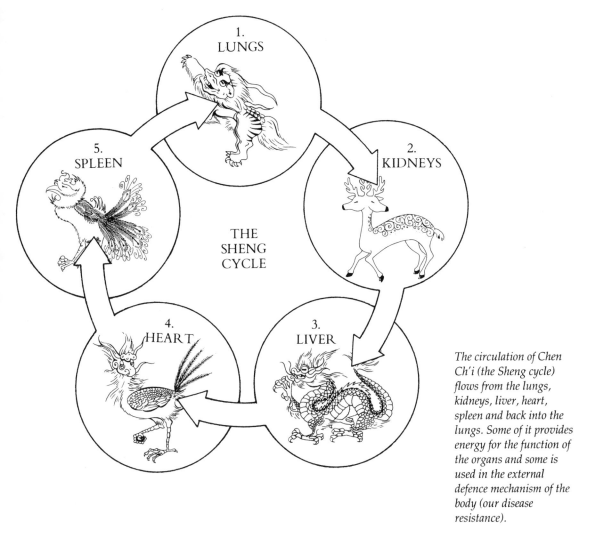

The circulation of Chen Ch'i (the Sheng cycle) flows from the lungs, kidneys, liver, heart, spleen and back into the lungs. Some of it provides energy for the function of the organs and some is used in the external defence mechanism of the body (our disease resistance).

the entire body through relaxed movement combined with breath control, without sweat, unaccustomed pressure or the high degree of discomfort that normally accompanies intense physical exertion.

Perhaps now is as good a time as any to look briefly at what certain Eastern and Western experts say about the science of breathing. World-famous yogi, Selvarajan Yesudian, writes in his book, *Yoga and Health* (Mandala, London, 1976):

OUR GREATEST MISTAKE: WE CANNOT BREATHE!

While we can survive for weeks without solid foods and several days without water, life without air is only possible for a few minutes. This shows that the connection between life and breath is the closest and that breathing is therefore the most important biological function of the organism. Every other activity of the body is closely connected with breathing. Breathing is of capital importance for our state of health, our emotional outlook and even for our longevity.

Civilised man does not know how to breathe! Our unnatural living conditions in modern city apartments and our cramped working conditions in factories and offices have resulted in our forgetting the rhythm of primitive breathing. Our stunted emotional life, the vacillation between passion and fear constrict our throats, and in the truest sense of the word, we do not dare to breathe deeply. The way in which children in this twentieth century breathe is scarcely enough for the merest vegetating. Their gasping is scarcely sufficient to keep them alive. How quickly this would change if people understood the ancient truth: only by the conscious regulation of our breathing can we achieve the resistance which assures us a long life free of sickness.

The equally famous Hindu, yogi Ramacharaka, states in his book *Science of Breath* (Yoga Publishing Company, USA):

BREATH IS LIFE

Breathing may be considered the most important of all of the functions of the body for, indeed, all the other functions depend upon it. Man may exist some time without eating; a shorter time without drinking; but without breathing his existence may be measured by a few minutes.

And not only is man dependent upon breath for life, but he is largely dependent upon correct habits of breathing for continued vitality and freedom from disease. An intelligent control of our breathing power will lengthen our days upon the earth by giving us increased vitality and

powers of resistance, and, on the other hand, unintelligent and careless
breathing will tend to shorten our days, by decreasing our vitality and
laying us open to disease.

The percentage of civilised men who breathe correctly is quite small,
and the result is shown in contracted chests and stooping shoulders,
and the terrible increase in diseases of the respiratory organs, including
that dread monster, consumption, 'the white scourge'. Eminent
authorities have stated that one generation of correct breathers would
regenerate the race, and disease would be so rare as to be looked upon
as a curiosity. Whether looked at from the standpoint of the Oriental
or Occidental, the connection between correct breathing and health is
readily seen and explained.

The Occidental teachings show that the physical health depends very
materially upon correct breathing. The Oriental teachers not only
admit that their Occidental brothers are right, but say that in addition
to the physical benefit derived from correct habits of breathing, man's
mental power, happiness, self-control, clear-sightedness, morals and
even his spiritual growth may be increased by an understanding of the
'Science of Breath'.

Such quotations could fill several volumes, being gathered from
the writings of many great thinkers and philosophers of every
nationality and from every part of the world throughout the ages.
There is a similarity among them all when it comes to the question of
breathing and its effect on our lives. Yet breathing has remained the
least considered, the least important of all aspects of physical and
psychological welfare in an age when we are desperately looking at
every conceivable angle for improved living and future survival. We
can only assume that because it is so easy to breathe 'normally', to
just let one breath follow another, that the idea of controlling it for the
benefit of our body rarely seems to be worth the effort. Unless, of
course, we have a specific reason to develop diaphragm-breathing, as
is necessary for singing,

The Chinese opera star for instance, is expected to keep up several
hours of non-stop 'singing' commentary without appearing to draw a
breath, the words and notes being linked endlessly together. To
cultivate the lung power, they practise by facing a wall, a few centimetres away from it, and never allowing the vibrations or echo of
their voice to die away.

To the Aboriginal people of Australia the didgeridoo is a sacred
tribal instrument. A hollow wooden tube up to 2 metres long (the
sound it gives is very like its name didgeridoooodidgeridooo-
didgeridooo), it must be played incessantly throughout a corroboree

(ritualistic dance) to keep away evil spirits who will return once it stops. It has no reeds or valve holes and, unlike the bagpipe, no goatskin or bladder of air to store a reserve while the player draws breath. The honour of playing the didgeridoo is handed down by the elders to a chosen few who are trained as boys. They are given a hollow reed to blow through and told to sit by the edge of a billabong (waterhole) with one end of the reed in their mouths and the other well below the surface, the idea being that the air bubbles blown from the reed never cease. By constant practice the boy learns to inhale whilst he is exhaling.

To a lesser degree, the saxophonist, trumpeter or any wind instrument player must learn to harness and use breath to its fullest advantage. Although you may never have blasted or squeezed your breath through any kind of instrument, it is reasonable to hope that, as the reader of this book, you have given the matter of breathing for health more thought than is customary.

If you are more than normally active, jog or walk regularly, play sport, attend a gym or exercise class, your aerobic (breath, heart and lung) capacity is probably stronger than if you did nothing. But that doesn't necessarily mean you use it to its best advantage or that you can't improve on it.

Unless you have been specifically taught deep-breathing techniques as part of a particular sport, like swimming or scuba diving, or for some special purpose such as Hatha Yoga or singing or playing wind instruments, you have probably never thought much about your breathing habits, lung capacity, diaphragm or oxygen intake — unless you have at some time been deprived of air, a traumatic experience that quickly puts the importance of breathing in its right perspective.

To find out just how ready you are to begin deep breathing exercises — whether you are in good shape to go straight into it or whether you should perhaps approach it slowly with gradual changes to your breathing habits — here are some suggestions. You have been breathing the way you do all your life, so increasing the length and depth of your inhalations and exhalations should be developed slowly and gently, in some cases even cautiously, and gradually built up.

The main thing to remember is that you have plenty of time, there is no hurry. The experience you are about to embark on can be of great value in your life, if it is accepted and persevered with. Begin by testing the length and depth of your in-breath and out-breath. Count silently in seconds or use the second hand of a clock or stopwatch. Do not drag air in noisily or hurriedly. If you find you tend to do this when taking a conscious breath there are basic Chi Kung methods to help you control it.

First, roll your tongue inwards, forming a cushion against the roof of your mouth. Close your teeth until they are gently touching and press the rolled cushion of your tongue firmly upward and forward until it is resting against the ridge of your upper jaw and comfortably filling the cavity of your closed mouth. By consciously tightening the tongue muscle, and at the same time tightening the rectum* you form a dam against the escape of Ch'i and at the same time guide the breath more directly through the nostrils. (As an alternative you may leave the tongue uncurled and press its tip firmly but comfortably against the back of the closed teeth.)

As you breathe in, allow the nostrils to flare slightly and concentrate on directing the air down the back of the throat until you can actually feel the coolness of its passage deeper and deeper — imagine it travelling down the spine rather than filling the lungs, being sure that your spine is perfectly upright. If you are a normal breather — one who is seldom conscious of inhalation and exhalation with little or no exercise, sporting activity or physical labour, your intake will be from 4 to 5 seconds, partially filling your lungs and going no further.

If you are a conscious breather, more aware of inhalation and exhalation — a regular exerciser, jogger, squash or tennis player, golfer, aerobic dancer or are involved in physical labour — your breath will be longer and deeper say, from 5 to 10 seconds, and more likely to penetrate to the diaphragm, in the region of the solar plexus.

If you are an athlete involved in training that calls for intense aerobic activity, as most sport does, your breath and lung capacity will be considerably more developed, but this does not necessarily mean that you are controlling that capacity to its fullest extent and getting the complete benefit of it. Should you by any chance be a trained singer or a trumpet player — someone who uses the breath to project sound — your breathing technique will be highly developed.

Whichever category you place yourself in, the aim is to slow down your in-breath and out-breath to say, a comfortable 30 to 40 seconds. This can increase to 60 seconds with practice. Your breath-holding capacity should more or less match the length of inhalation and exhalation. An excellent way to measure, control and develop this is to follow the 'yogic walk', suggested on page 196. After a while you will be able to breathe in for 20 or 30 leisurely paces, hold your breath and allow it to circulate for 20 to 30 paces (or counts), then exhale over 20 to 30 paces. Don't hurry it or become impatient. Aim for, say, 12 paces (or counts) in, 12 paces hold, 12 paces out, and take it from there.

As so many of us spend more time than we would like behind the

---

* Conscious tensing of the anal sphincter during breathing exercise is considered not only to help contain the Ch'i, but also to benefit or guard against haemorrhoidal conditions and strengthen the prostate gland.

wheel of a car, a variation of this can be practised while driving, just by counting your breaths.

The other aspect to concentrate on is silence. Regulate the flow of air-energy into your body until it is completely soundless. This takes time but it can be achieved and it is an excellent method of breath control. Tell yourself you are in a strict Kung Fu training session and the Sifu is walking among the class, his sensitive ear cocked for the slightest hint of sound and one hundred knuckle press-ups for the breather he detects.

This does not mean that if you cannot completely silence your breath you cannot continue. Your early efforts will probably find the sound of your own breath impossible to suppress. So begin by asking someone else at home if they can hear you breathe — strive at least to control it until it cannot be heard by another, no matter how closely they listen. At the same time test the depth of your breathing by placing the palm of your hand lightly on the stomach just below the sternum and feel for the breath to rise and fall in this area rather than the chest. If you cannot feel it yourself ask someone else to check it for you.

The Passages of Ch'i

The network of Ch'i channels throughout the body direct the life force into every organ and extremity. In Chinese medicine these passages are known as meridians, Ch'i channels and/or collaterals. They are seen as conduits of energy, an essential system that links the superficial (skin and flesh) with the internal system of the trunk (muscle and bone), that joins the upper and lower parts of the body, co-ordinates the limbs and connects the solid organs (heart, liver, kidney) to the hollow organs (lungs, intestines, spleen, gall and urinary bladder).

These passages are not to be confused with blood vessels, veins, arteries or nerves. They are special routes that the Chinese believe form the circuitry of human performance, both physical and mental. The main channels (jing) are the major pipelines of supply throughout the body while the collaterals are the branch lines, tapping into the main source, distributing Ch'i energy (oxygen) and connecting the whole.

The Chinese also believe that when a fault or breakdown of this intricate circuitry occurs, no matter how minor, the free flow of Ch'i is impeded and illness or disease will result; that if the Ch'i channels and collaterals are kept open and the flow of energy increased through a combination of breathing therapy, exercise and basic nutrition, human performance knows no bounds. A theory that is best seen in evidence through the practice of dynamic Chi Kung (martial arts) and in the remarkable effect upon health through quiescent Chi Kung (breathing exercises for healing).

Because these meridians are not normally recognised by Western medical science, they are only shown here as a matter of interest rather than medical fact. However, if there is any credibility in acupuncture — perhaps the oldest of all Chinese healing methods — then, the meridians are the key to its 360 vital points.

Dating as far back as 1500 BC, the history of acupuncture is not well documented, but the belief that vital energy — the life force known as Ch'i — travels these invisible meridians is as widely accepted in China today as it was thousands of years ago.

As different to explain or prove as the phenomena of Ch'i itself, the following translation from a book on Chinese Chi Kung compiled by China's leading masters, gives the following explanation: 'When the mind is quiescent and void, true Ch'i will be at your command. If one keeps a sound mind, danger of disease will turn to safety.'

These are the words of the Yellow Emperor's Canon of Internal Medicine, written in 2597 BC. So, the source of true Ch'i is closely related to the emptying of the mind — to be relaxed, content and natural. In the words of modern medicine, this would put the cerebral cortex into a 'special' quiescent state, regulate the central nervous system and adjust its disorders. Thus it can be seen that a quiet mind is the first precondition for promoting the free flow of internal energy ... true Ch'i. The *Yellow Emperor's Canon* also said:

If you take the whole world in your heart, have a good command of Yin and Yang, breathe the essential air and keep a sound mind, your muscles will function smoothly, your organs will remain young and you will live as long as the earth exists.

One of the most important principles of traditional Chinese medicine and the concept of Chi Kung, is to start with the body as a whole: to regulate the entire system, to diagnose and treat the condition on the basis of overall analysis rather than inflexible symptomatic treatment.

Considering these opinions have been steadfastly adhered to over the millennia, it is not surprising that more and more Western medical institutions are beginning to apply the holistic approach to prevention and cure; that an increasing number of people in our society are investigating the alternatives open to them for improved health and wellbeing.

The Chinese principle of the meridians that channel the Ch'i — the power within — is perhaps the hardest to conceive but the most dynamic to apply.

There are twelve main channels that regulate the Yin (solid) organs and the Yang (hollow) organs. The six Yin channels travel the interior laterals connecting lungs, pericardium, heart, spleen, liver and kidney and hold the hollow organs in place. The six Yang channels travel the exterior laterals connecting the large intestine, the triple warmer, the small intestine, the stomach, the gall bladder, the urinary bladder and hold the solid organs in place.

THE TWELVE CHANNELS OF CH'I

YIN CHANNELS	YANG CHANNELS	PASSAGE — UPPER BODY
Solid organs hold hollow organs through interior laterals	Hollow organs hold solid organs through exterior laterals.	Parts of the body the Ch'i channels pass through
The lung-hand channel	The large intestine-hand channel	Anterior line
The pericardium-hand channel	The triple warmer-hand channel	Midline
The heart-hand Channel	The small intestine-hand channel	Posterior
YIN CHANNELS	YANG CHANNELS	PASSAGE — LOWER BODY
The spleen-foot channel	The stomach-foot channel	Anterior line-midline
The liver-foot channel	The gall bladder-foot channel	Midline-anterior line
The kidney-foot channel	The urinary bladder-foot channel	Posterior line

The triple warmer is an obscure but vital organ in Chinese medicine best described by Western doctors as the heart governor. The triple warmer (or heater) controls the process of circulation — respiratory, digestive and excretory, which in turn regulate body temperature.

The Ch'i channels are further separated into hand and foot meridians — three Yin hand channels, three Yin foot channels; three Yang hand channels and three Yang foot channels.

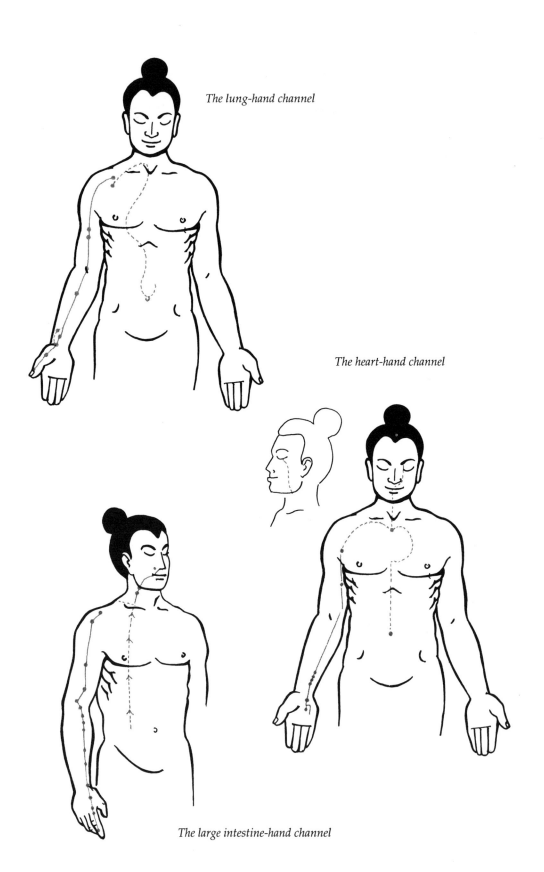

The lung-hand channel

The heart-hand channel

The large intestine-hand channel

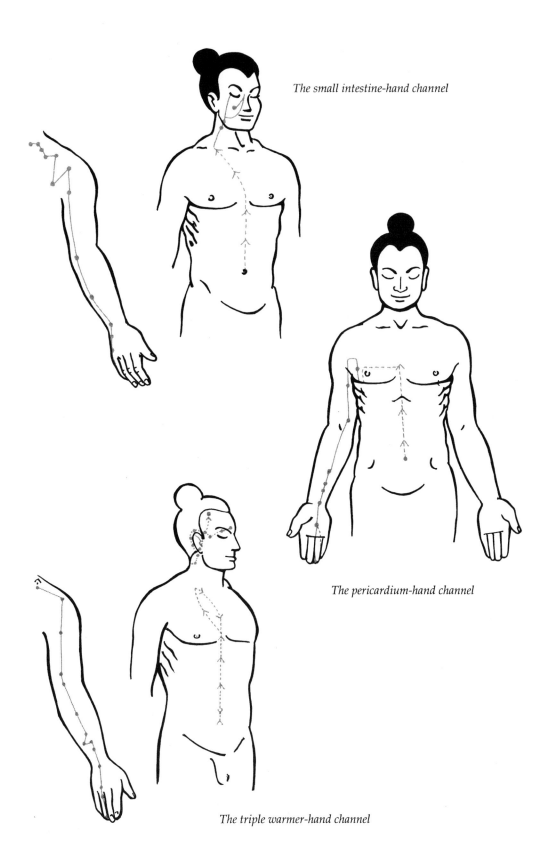

The small intestine-hand channel

The pericardium-hand channel

The triple warmer-hand channel

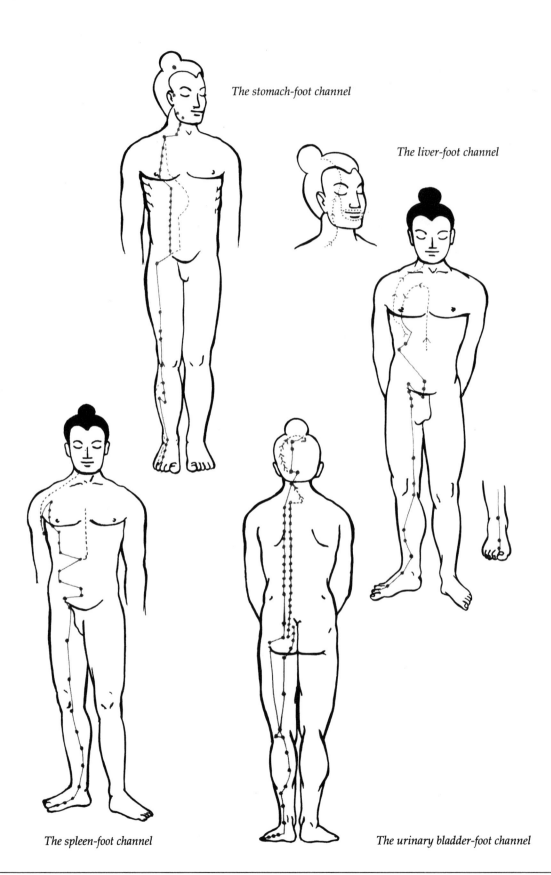

The stomach-foot channel

The liver-foot channel

The spleen-foot channel

The urinary bladder-foot channel

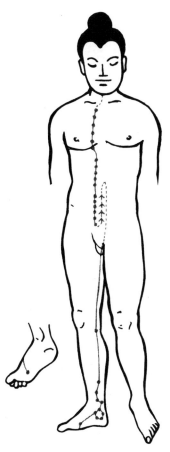

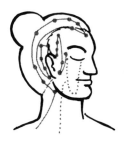

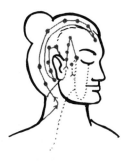

The gall bladder-foot channel

The kidney-foot channel

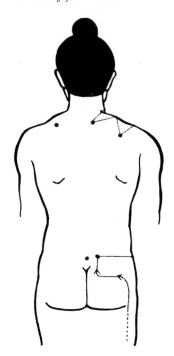

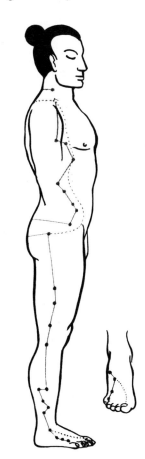

STILLING THE MIND

氣

An element of Chi Kung essential to success is complete concentration. The Chinese call it 'quietude'; we may see it as tranquillity, serenity, or even meditation. Concentration is the first stage of meditation, the contemplation of a single thought or vision which if held long enough induces a state of self-communication that excludes all else. The purpose of concentration is to close the mind to all outside interference in order to be at peace with oneself — not so easy to achieve in today's world and the pace we are expected to keep up.

The mind, said the Chinese sages, is like a running tiger — not easy to catch, slow down and tame. Or, like a runaway horse bolting without direction to its own destruction, it must be reined in, gentled and mastered. Quietude is probably one of the most difficult conditions to achieve in the often overpowering pressures of today's world.

There are simple methods that can improve the powers of concentration significantly. They are not suggested as types of meditation (far deeper trance-like states best left to the experienced teacher), but purely as methods of relaxation.

The object of concentration is twofold:

The visual ... *what you see.*
The mental ... *what you think.*

If the eyes wander, so does the mind. Choose an object in front of you, half close your eyes and gaze at it steadily. It may be a leaf, the branch of a shrub, a distant tree, a landmark on the horizon, the house across the road or a cloud formation.

Focus your eyes upon it as you would a camera lens until you are aware of nothing else within your field of vision. Let no movement or intrusion distract you from it; if it does, your concentration is broken and you must refocus.

Your mental concentration should fix on the upper and then lower Tan T'ien (see diagrams). First, the upper point, dead centre between the eyebrows. Imagine it as a pinpoint of white light, a miniature sun, fixed in place by your willpower. Allow it to sink with the intake of your breath to the lower Tan T'ien, that point directly below your navel in line with the base of the spine. Hold it there with your willpower. Imagine you have used your own will to locate and shift your energy from the brain to your centre of gravity.

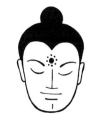

Position of the upper Tan T'ien.

If this sounds strange and unnecessary to you, think of it this way. We often conjure things up in our mind's eye, or imagination. Some have a stronger imagination than others, but we all have one. We can use it to stimulate our emotions, consciously and unconsciously. In most of us it was stronger in infancy and childhood before we learned the difference between fact and fantasy, and began to demand explanation, logic or proof.

When we were very young, the world of the unreal was usually preferable to the real. We could retreat into the realms of giants and fairies, elves and pixies, all the hidden places of our own perception of wonderland any time we felt like it. For most of us except those referred to as 'simple', who for some reason remain childlike, reality asserts itself and fantasy fades, put into perspective by development into adulthood.

It is never too late to recapture imagination, in fact it often returns with old age, when once again, as though tired of the world, we have discovered we seek refuge in fantasy. If it seems that too much emphasis is put upon this aspect of Chi Kung, remember it plays a vital role. Without the ability to imagine Ch'i, which is impossible to see, to locate the Tan T'ien in your mind's eye, to imagine the healing journey of air down through the body to that hidden powerhouse in your belly, your Ch'i will not learn to flow.

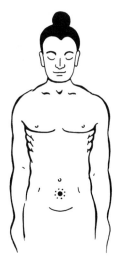

Position of the lower Tan T'ien.

As always, there is a Chinese saying, proverb or poem to illustrate it. In fact there are many. This poem is taken from the famous Tao Te Ching:

> *Because the eye gazes but can catch no glimpse of it,*
> *it is called elusive.*
> *Because the ear listens but cannot hear it,*
> *it is called rarefied.*
> *Because the hand feels for it but cannot find it,*
> *it is called the infinitesimal.*
> *Its rising brings no light;*
> *its sinking no darkness.*
> *It is called Ch'i.*

So, indulge in a little fantasy but do not let it run riot. Rein it in, focus it and for the period of your practice let all your imaginative powers reside in that one precious, all-powerful point of light. Then, learn to control it. To materialise it in that exact spot 5 centimetres below the navel, until with time you will begin to feel its glow, feel its healing power radiate from there to whichever area of the body you wish to direct it.

If you find your mind needs something else to dwell upon, memorise a poem, something really pleasant to contemplate. Repeat it, analyse it, become lost in it in the same way that the yogi repeats a mantra. Poetry or prose has always played an important part in the finer aspects of Chinese culture. The conjuring up of the sublime state, no matter how out of place in modern surroundings can be a great aid to total relaxation.

EATING, DRINKING, SMOKING AND CH'I
氣

Most serious exercise routines or forms of health improvement call
for some kind of diet restriction or change in eating habits. This one
does not necessarily do so. What, when and how much you eat is far
less critical to a healthy system than an unhealthy one, and improved
breathing is far more important than a careful diet. That is to say, a
person practising Pa Tuan Tsin diligently is less likely to suffer the ill-
effects of eating unwisely. Of course, the proper foods are of major
importance to physical well-being, but a well-tuned state of health
and a built-in resistance is better equipped to cope than a slack and
sickly one.

Regular exercise of the right kind, taken at the right time and in
the right amount, is the best antidote to illness. We know it is not as
simple as it sounds. Life has spurred most of us from a walk to a trot,
from a canter to a gallop, so that it's not that easy to slow down, stop,
think and act. Unless of course, we are prepared to adjust our whole
pattern of life: change our job to give us more time, pore over
dietitians' charts, herbal tonics and the dos and don'ts of health
books that point out with frightening candour, the things we have
been doing wrong for most of our lives.

Few of us are prepared to grasp the nettle to that extent. That is
not to say that for those with the strength of purpose to discover and
enjoy 'health foods' or even a vegetarian diet, careful eating is not of
tremendous benefit. It is, but a healthy system comes first. Counting
calories and cholesterol and balancing proteins may not be as vital to
a long and energetic existence as some would have us think.

As a general rule, the strongest and fittest among us are those who work outdoors. But the number of such people is diminishing in the face of rapid takeover of air-conditioned, computerised, mechanical labour-savers. I once worked with a lumberjack named Cauliflower Sid, who ate little but tinned cauliflower, as the ever-growing mountain of tins outside his tent testified. But he also felled more timber than men half his age. He was seventy-two and died at eighty-two after falling from a galloping horse. You will often find such renegades battling on into old age without so much as a bellyache, while their more cautious counterparts behind a desk develop ulcers, headaches, varicose veins and haemorrhoids.

With the greatest respect for health foods, men like Cauliflower Sid have probably never heard of 'we are what we eat', otherwise they would all have gone to an untimely grave under a monument of empty cans, bacon grease, dried meat, hard tack and bangers 'n' mash ... not to mention strong tobacco and hard liquor.

Consider the huge work force of the Third World. Throughout the East you will find middle-aged to elderly Chinese women trotting up and down the plants of building sites all day balancing baskets of sand and cement; Indians, Indonesians, Filipinos and Malays labouring ten to sixteen hour days — all on a bowl of rice, a chunk of dried fish or meat and a spoonful of green vegetables if they're lucky. They smoke cheap cheroots, drink cheap booze, gamble half the night, bear many children and usually call it a day in their eighties, with a roomful of respectful great-grandchildren paying for a festive send-off.

All this should indicate that physical toil is nature's exercise that all of us were built to perform, and it helps greatly when it comes to avoiding the results of inadequate or unwise diet. How does this knowledge help us in our own situation, surrounded as most of us are by a convenient variety of highly refined processed, frozen, dehydrated supermarket edibles?

If we are honest with ourselves, we probably accept that a dramatic change in our eating habits is unlikely to last. If there are certain things you really enjoy eating and that you have always eaten, giving them up altogether may not seem worth the sacrifice. Perhaps it isn't. With the tremendous research and millions of words written on the subject of 'eating for health', we all have a fair idea of what we should and shouldn't put into our stomachs. Many of us have been through the stage of the balanced health food diet; trundled off to the bulk store for our ration of brans, grains, dried fruit, nuts and nature foods. Who hasn't been frightened by the suggestion that we have been slowly but surely poisoning ourselves for most of our lifetime! But how many of us have stuck with a serious attempt to revise our daily menu? It's like smoking and drinking. It just isn't as simple as that! A sizzling plate of bacon and eggs with white toast and black coffee can be hard to reject for a bowl of wheat germ and raisins.

So we compromise and cut down, often only when we are advised to do so by a doctor. Sometimes, gradual change is far better than sudden denial. You don't confuse your insides or confound your palate by stopping a life-long custom.

If we are not prepared to take a course in mathematics in order to compute the exact measurements and balance accurate combinations, there is always a simple formula:

> *Eat less meat and more fish and fowl.*
> *Eat less protein and more carbohydrate.*
> *Eat less processed food and more raw vegetables.*
> *Eat less animal fats and more vegetable oil.*
> *Eat less white sugar and sweets and replace with honey and raw sugar.*
> *Eat less white flour and biscuits and more fresh fruit.*
> *Eat less refined cereals and more roughage.*

Now, to drinking. If we really want to know what alcohol does to our insides, there are many books on that disturbing subject. We don't need to be told that alcohol and serious exercise do not go together. One of the first warnings of Chin Wu is that of instant dismissal if the faintest whiff of alcohol is detected before a practice session. Refreshment during training is restricted to a large kettle of hot water or hot green tea (Ching Cha) from which students help themselves during training breaks (cold drinks are also forbidden).

What a person drinks in off-training time is his/her own affair, but he/she is strongly advised to stop taking liquor and never to drink anything ice-cold when hot. As with eating, it is the individual's choice and decision. Quite obviously, to quit entirely is best for the rehabilitation of the inner self. But again, let's be realistic. It doesn't matter why a person needs a drink or how many are needed to reach the desired effect. Be it relief from anxiety or depression, downright escapism, forced merriment, riotous behaviour or some good reason to celebrate, a drinking person is unlikely to stop for the promise of Pa Tuan Tsin or any other promise. At least not for long.

There is one very effective method of counteracting your intake and breaking down its harmful effects. It is not only a reconditioner of the liver and kidneys, where most harm is done by prolonged drinking, it is a health aid in itself and dates back as far as the origins of Wu Shu, although variations of it have long been practised all over the world with varying degrees of faith. It is the simple process of drinking a certain amount of pure water under certain conditions and at a certain time, known to the Chinese as water therapy.

Rather than attempt an explanation of my own, the following is a fairly faithful, if quaint, translation from an original Chinese document, in turn translated from a paper published by the Japanese Sickness Association in 1975. It turned up in Manila and copies were handed out to Chin Wu pupils with strong recommendations for its application during early morning practice of Pa Tuan Tsin.

This is a Chinese translated copy of Water Therapy which was taken from a paper written by a Japanese author whose name is not known to me. I found the salutary and curative effects of this therapy not only by my personal experience, but also by those who know the treatment and were applying it without any let-up. I am inspired to translate this Chinese copy into English with the aim of giving it to those who have not come across this knowledge of God-given therapy, especially to the poor who cannot afford modern medication. This therapy cures at absolutely no expense except that of our faith and perseverance.

The paper goes on to repeat a story which is reputed to have taken place long ago, and was apparently passed on by a very old but robust Chinese peasant. Some Chin Wu instructors, more from romantic imagination, I suspect, than from evidence, placed the events at 'more than a thousand years' ago. The full account is far too long and flowery to include here, but the following is a condensed version:

For a long time I had been ill. I was unable to perform the smallest tasks. For me the fields and streams, the trees on the mountain, the plumage of the peacock had lost their colour. Day was night and night was day. Grasshoppers did not sing, nor linnets. No flower opened. Then, a man came to the door of my hut and asked for rice. He was old, he said, but his body was young and he journeyed for the love of journeying and lived for the love of living. I gave him rice and he cut all my wood in a very short time, also mending the shingles of my roof. Before he left he told me this: 'Tonight, eat nothing for your supper but fruit. In the morning as soon as you arise, go to the well and fill a bucket. Do not wash or eat but breathe deeply the early morning air and drink one gallon of pure water as you watch the sun come up. Do this every day of your life and you will never grow old. All sickness will be banished and you will find new life.' Then he went on his way, strongly along the path.

Next morning I did as he had told me to. At first I found discomfort to drink so much. Many times I drained the cup. Many times I urinated and cleared my bowels. I felt a dizziness but still I drank. My conjee that morning tasted more delicious than ever before. After one week

I could drink all the water easily. I urinated only twice, my motions were normal and my head was clear. I quickly became well again and I have never been ill since, not even with cold or fever. This happened thirty years ago when I was forty. Everyday, I have taken the water without exception and everyday is new to me and better than the one that went before. Now I live for the love of life and journey for the love of journeying. I tell this story to all who will listen.

That is the gist of the document that created so much interest in the Chin Wu School in 1975. The writer goes on to say:

Such claims for the drinking of water seem unbelievable and inconceivable, but facts prove it to be reliable and recommendable. Drinking sufficient quantities of water at one time renders the colon more effective in forming more fresh blood, known in medical terms as hematopoiesis.

This is made possible by the function of the mucosa folds found in the colon and intestine. These folds absorb the nutrients from food taken by our bodies and turn them into new blood.

Due to insufficient exercise of the colonic tract, man feels exhausted, becomes sick and finds his ailments hard to cure. Adult human beings have colons (or large intestines) eight feet long, capable of absorbing the nutrients taken by us several times a day. This nutrition is completely absorbed by the mucosa folds which in turn prevent or cure our ailments and are considered a principal power in the improvement of our health. Water therapy completely flushes this vital system in regular cycles, thoroughly cleansing the mucosa folds where dangerous waste otherwise gathers and remains.

In other words, applying water therapy will make us healthier and prolong our mortal lives.

The full claims of this unusual document are, of course, open to a great deal of speculation, certainly on the question of quantity. It is probably true to say that too much water can wash out vital nutrients along with impurities. But the simple fact that no other liquid is known to be more widely beneficial or totally essential than plain water cannot be disputed. It is not only a reconditioner of the liver and kidneys, where most damage is done by overindulgence, it is a health aid in itself. Plain, unadulterated water is as free and available to most people as oxygen. We have always known water to be good for us — which is probably why we stop drinking it as soon as we can when we are kids. We seem to associate it with washing our necks and invasion of that very private territory behind the ears.

Drinking regular quantities of fresh, cool water by choice is fairly unexciting to some and its lack of popularity is not hard to understand when we consider the competition it has. The drinking tap is surrounded by so many persuasive alternatives. Even forgetting coffee, tea, soft drinks, the addictive everyday beverages we are more or less forced to consume, there are multitudes of 'health drinks', flavoured and preserved milk combinations, canned fruit juices, bottled essences, powdered mixtures ... so many things to flavour your water that the thought of drinking it on its own seems decidedly old-fashioned. Many of us go to our final resting place having never been closer to a regular water intake than cleaning our teeth and swallowing pills.

If you decide to try water therapy — in whatever quantity you find acceptable — it is vitally important that you do not miss a morning and therefore break the cycle. After three or four weeks, you will find it as much a part of your ablutions as visiting the bathroom.

Do *not* put the water in the fridge. Drink it warm rather than very cold — boiled, distilled or filtered rather than straight from the tap. If you believe in nothing else, you will find that you can take your usual intake of alcohol with less effect, hangovers will be a thing of the past and you will know that your liver and kidneys are being thoroughly taken care of. *Water therapy is not an essential part of Pa Tuan Tsin* but the drinking of some water, however little it may be, is strongly recommended during the exercise period.

Smoking cigarettes, cigars, pipe tobacco or anything else you habitually draw into your lungs, cannot possibly help in the development of any form of respiratory exercise and health improvement: the cutting down or cutting out most certainly will.

As with alcohol and junk foods, it is a question of degree. It is also an undeniable fact that some people happily smoke their lives away to a ripe old age while others choke it away long before they should. There will always be the popular argument among heavy smokers that they could give up smoking, walk outside and get run over by a bus or that a lungful of polluted city air, diesel fumes, chemical waste, factory smoke, jet vapour, not to mention nuclear fallout and regular doses of carbon monoxide, could do them more harm than a six-month supply of tobacco. Printed health warnings and the ban on television advertising don't do much to convince a confirmed smoker. Even hideous films of a heavy smoker's lungs will at best make them sweat a little — and fumble for a nerve stick afterwards.

In these days of high stress points and low resistance, increased anxiety factors and mounting psychological strain, it is not surprising to find the number of people lighting up greater than the number giving up. So, as with the excesses of tasty food and good liquor, it is pointless suggesting that you cut it down or cut it out. You know by now what your two packs a day are doing to you and you don't need anyone to remind you — the hacking and barking you do each morning over the washbasin does that, so does the taste in your mouth and the shortness of your breath.

What may make you think twice is the difficulty you will find when trying to prolong your breath intake. A non-smoker can quite quickly develop inhalation and exhalation of thirty seconds plus. If you are a heavy smoker, ten seconds may well be your limit. Almost certainly, if you take Pa Tuan Tsin seriously, you will automatically begin to cut down. First, you will avoid your early morning drag in preparation for exercise: the exercises themselves prohibit smoking during practice. You are unlikely to feel like one directly afterwards and may be well on your way to the office or halfway through the morning before you find yourself reaching for the cigarettes.

When Pa Tuan Tsin has become a regular part of your routine, say in the second or third month, the effects of increased oxygen and controlled breathing will prove so much more beneficial to peace of mind and bodily wellbeing that you may finally give up altogether.

THE TIME AND PLACE

Now that we know a little about the exercises and the dos and don'ts that go with them so far as eating, drinking and smoking are concerned, there are one or two other simple but very important questions to consider. First, what is the best time to practise Pa Tuan Tsin?

The ideal time for breathing exercises, the Masters say, is between 1 a.m. and 3 a.m. This might have been fine for the Shaolin monks, but they didn't have colour television and probably went to bed at sundown. Also, most of their true rest came from advanced meditation. They had reached a state of Ch'i that called for no more than three to five hours sleep.

To bring things up to date: unless you are having difficulty with sleep (in which case, fifteen minutes or so of breathing exercises can do wonders), early morning is by far the best time (as early as your daily demands allow), or second best, late evening.

First, for morning breathers. We all differ in our waking habits — some are fresh and energetic while others take an hour to get moving. Whichever you are, as your enthusiasm grows with progress, you will find it becomes easier to rise early, feeling refreshed and eager to exercise at 5 a.m. When the world is still asleep, nothing could be better. If not, as close to it as you can manage without destroying your whole routine.

The benefits of the early morning are obvious. The air, whether you are in Pittsburg or Putney, is at its best and distraction is at its lowest. So, for early morning breathers the ideal time is on rising, as early as possible, and finishing in time to allow half an hour before eating and fifteen minutes before bathing. *Do not shower or bath for at least fifteen minutes after finishing your exercise. When you do, make it a warm or hot one, never ice-cold. Allow at least half an hour before breakfast. Never nibble or sip during exercise unless it's cool to warm water or clear Chinese green tea.* (You can buy 'Ching Cha' from any Chinese store and many supermarkets.)

If circumstances make it easier for you to be an evening breather, your best time is an hour or so after dinner or within a half hour before going to bed.

On rising, drink two or three glasses of pure water; visit toilet. Do not wash thoroughly, just sluice the face and solar plexus with cold water. Warm-up exercises for fifteen minutes. Brief rest. *Do not sit down.* Breathing exercises for fifteen minutes. Brief rest: ten-minute walk (or just move around). *Do not sit down.* Prepare for shower or bath. Eat breakfast.

THE IDEAL ROUTINE

The length of time you spend on Pa Tuan Tsin will increase with your progress. As a beginner, you should slot twenty to thirty minutes into your day.

The best place to practise Pa Tuan Tsin depends on location and surroundings. The essentials are freedom from interruption and any form of distraction. If you have a garden, select a spot in it. If you know of a place within easy reach, a park, a field, a beach, aim for it. If you live in a high-rise building, the open window of your bedroom with the door locked will do nicely.

It is easy to imagine how simple it was for the monks of Shaolin in the scented gardens of their mountain retreat, watching the sun rise like a gong. Nothing bigger than the birds and bugs to contend with. What about early traffic? Kids? The neighbour's radio? All you can do is find the quietest and most private place your particular world allows ... the best available air and the least chance of distraction. *Use the same spot every day, facing the same direction.* Fix your attention on some object and don't lose it ... a flower, a leaf, a distant cloud, anything that is quiet and natural.

> *Quiet and private as possible.*
> *Best available air.*
> *Same spot and direction.*
> *Concentrate on one pleasant object.*
> *Rid the mind of all else.*

If you follow this routine without breaking it for the first month, you will find the mind and body begin to work as one, the exercises will seem to take control and your mind will go along for the ride. It is a wonderful feeling of true relaxation and growing strength. Two additional rules which only you can insist upon are consistency and mental attitude. Consistent practice and positive thinking.

THE IDEAL SITUATION

For the quickest and most definite results Pa Tuan Tsin should be practised every day, and this is what you should aim for. If you feel at first that this is too much, begin with every other day, or even two to three times a week will do. Your own progress will increase your stamina, your enthusiasm and your frequency. Once a day-to-day pattern is achieved, try not to break it. It is not advisable to perform Pa Tuan Tsin in any state of anxiety, distress or excitement. It is better not to try. You will know if the disturbance is stronger than your will in the first five minutes. Don't persevere. If you find your thoughts competing unsuccessfully with your exercise, *stop. Don't fight or work at it.* The essence of Pa Tuan Tsin is quietude and relaxation.

WHAT TO WEAR

Whatever is loose-fitting and comfortable is the correct clothing for the practice of Pa Tuan Tsin. A tracksuit is fine if it is cold, pyjamas are ideal if you are indoors. An old pair of pyjama trousers and a T-shirt will suffice if the weather is mild and you practise outside. It is not advisable to practise stripped to the waist until you are well advanced. Initially, you may sweat, which can leave you liable to chill.

Never exercise with a leather or stiff belt, this not only interferes with breathing but can be dangerous to internal organs, especially when practising deep bends. A sash, old scarf, necktie or any sort of soft cord is comfortable without restricting freedom of movement. Footwear should be soft and preferably without heels, rubber soles or any non-slip soles. Avoid plastic. The traditional black, elastic-sided Chinese slippers are best, easily found in Chinese stores. Tennis or track shoes or perhaps an old pair of carpet slippers is a good alternative. Remove your wristwatch, neck chain, rings or any other accessories you may be in the habit of wearing. If your hair is long, the wearing of a sweatband around the forehead is a good idea.

You are ready to start your first Pa Tuan Tsin practice session. You may or may not have found it necessary to practise the simple deep breathing exercises mentioned on page 87 in order to increase your lung capacity.

The demonstration in the illustrated section that follows have been separated into four parts: 1 Stances; 2 The Warm-up; 3 Pa Tuan Tsin; 4 Extra Exercises.

Remember:

PATIENCE

DISCIPLINE

FORTITUDE

CONFIDENCE

INTRODUCTORY CHI KUNG EXERCISES

Here are five preliminary breathing exercises as taught in Chinese breath therapy clinics to help the student or patient to 'walk before you can run', to apply the basic principles of Chi Kung in simple form before going further. Approach the exercises in the following way:

Apply the imagination to locate the upper and lower Tan T'ien as suggested previously. Enter the state of quietude. Concentrate on the elimination of all extraneous sound and vision until you have no sense of position or weight. A gentle drifting sensation, conscious yet unconscious, aware but unaware until a state of tranquillity is reached with complete relaxation of body and mind, a total harmony.

This can be helped by counting your breathing, not unlike the old European practice of counting sheep to help fall asleep. Silently count each breath in and out up to 100, taking care to suppress the sound.

Focus and remain focused regardless of distraction. Recite poetry in the mind.

Spend a week or two with these very basic introductory breathing exercises until you really feel an improvement in the depth, flow and regulation of your breath and are confident enough of your patience and tolerance.

These introductory exercises are very convenient to practise in bed, relaxing in the garden, even watching TV — in any few moments to yourself anywhere, anytime. They are also ideal for those who are not accustomed to regular fitness routines, in poor health, recovering from illness or injury, heavy smokers intent on cutting down or giving up and for the elderly. It is recommended that an understanding of breath control be first explored with these introductory exercises before going on to advanced or dynamic Chi Kung.

The standing, sitting and lying down postures are designed to nourish your Ch'i. Known as 'lutrinsic nourishing exercise' there are some very basic rules to follow for each of the stationary postures.

♦ Clear the mind by repeating words or sentences (silently) that suggest calm and tranquillity.

♦ Be aware of the position of the tongue.

♦ Concentrate on the flow of Ch'i from the upper Tan T'ien between the eyes, directing it to the lower Tan T'ien, 5 centimetres below the navel.

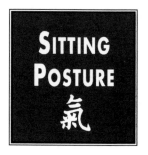

SITTING POSTURE
氣

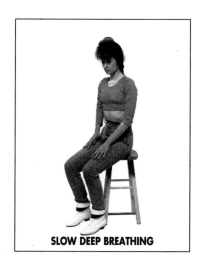

SLOW DEEP BREATHING

Seat yourself on a hard stool or chair — feet about 20 centimetres apart and pointed forwards in line with your knees. Allow your head to rest slightly forwards, your chest and shoulders relaxed without drooping forwards. Relax your hands and place them on your knees. Half close your eyes, or fully close them if you feel more comfortable. Allow the tension to drain away, shut out extraneous noise, concentrate on nothing but the rhythm and quality of your breathing.

Breathe slowly and deeply, willing the Ch'i to travel downwards to the lower Tan T'ien. Imagine the purifying air, energised by your life force.

Hold this position for as long as is comfortable. With patient practice, increase the length of time you can hold the position. Stop if you feel yourself falling.

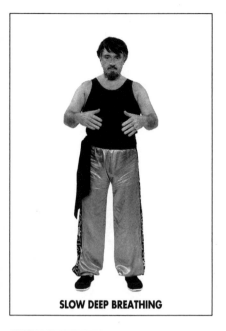

SLOW DEEP BREATHING

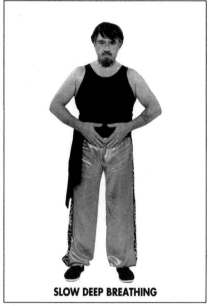

SLOW DEEP BREATHING

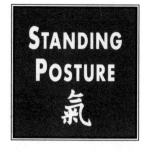

STEP 1 ▲

This exercise is sometimes called 'The Tree' or 'The Sacred Tree' because it resembles the embracing of a tree.

Stand straight with your feet slightly (20 centimetres) apart, toes pointing forwards. Your knees should be slightly bent as your arms are raised to lower chest level (to embrace the imaginary tree). Your hands should be relaxed and your fingers slightly curled inwards (as though holding an imaginary ball in each hand).

Breathe slowly and deeply, directing the flow of your Ch'i downwards. Concentrate only on the age and strength of the tree, the power of the sap which gives life to its limbs and the power of your own Ch'i.

Hold this position as long as is comfortable. With patient practice, increase the length of time you can hold the position.

STEP 2 ▲

A variation to The Tree is to 'Touch the Tan T'ien'.

Stand as in Step 1. Sink your shoulders comfortably and move your head and neck gently to rid the area of all tension. Allow your hands to hang loosely at your sides. Slowly raise them until the palms are pressed lightly on the abdomen and relaxed fingertips are 'touching' the area of Tan T'ien below the navel.

Breathe slowly and deeply, imagining the Ch'i gathering under your fingertips, the palms rising and falling with the movement of your regular, unhurried breathing.

Hold this position as long as is comfortable. With patient practice, increase the length of time you can hold the position.

LYING POSTURE — SIDEWAYS 氣

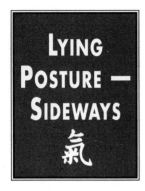

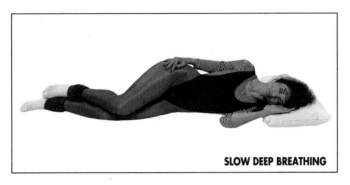

SLOW DEEP BREATHING

Lie down on the floor or on a firm bed or couch, head on a pillow, slightly forwards, back slightly bent. Place your lower hand on the pillow close to your face (palm upwards). Stretch your upper arm down the body to its full extent until your palm and outstretched fingers are resting naturally on your upper thigh. Stretch your lower leg fully but comfortably and keep your upper leg slightly bent.

Breathe slowly and deeply, willing the Ch'i downward to the lower Tan T'ien. Clear the mind of all else but this invigorating passage.

Hold as long as is comfortable and with patient practice increase the length of time you can hold the position. This form of intrinsically nourishing breathing may send you to sleep.

LYING POSTURE — ON THE BACK 氣

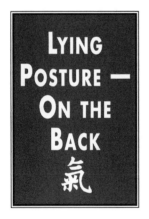

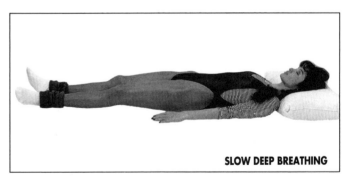

SLOW DEEP BREATHING

Lie flat on the floor or on a firm bed or couch with your head resting comfortably on a firm, shallow pillow (the harder the better). Stretch your arms full length down your body, fingers comfortably outstretched, palms facing downwards. Stretch your legs fully but without tension, your heels should be touching each other and your toes relaxed.

Breathe slowly and deeply in a steady rhythm. Concentrate on nothing but the circulation of your Ch'i.

Hold this position as long as is comfortable. With patient practice, increase the length of time you can hold the position.

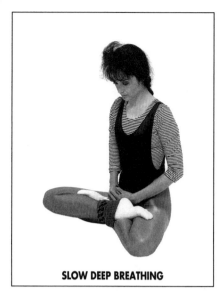

SLOW DEEP BREATHING

This familiar posture of meditation will be very well known to those who have studied yoga or forms of meditation. It is the classic pose of serenity as practised by Gautama Buddha and named after the flower of tranquillity. It won't be immediately comfortable but will get easier with practice. Your ability to sit for long periods in the lotus position will depend upon your flexibility.

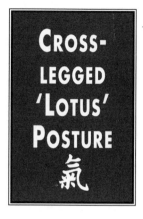

CROSS-LEGGED 'LOTUS' POSTURE
氣

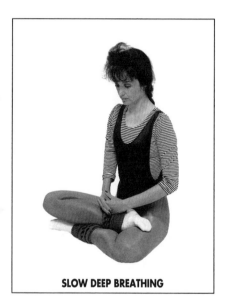

SLOW DEEP BREATHING

◀ **S T E P   2**

If you decide to practise this exercise, the half-lotus (not quite so hard on the joints) is enough until you become more flexible. Keep your spine straight, shoulders and chest relaxed, head slightly forward.

Breathe slowly and deeply, concentrate on the soundlessness of your breathing, imagine the flow of your Ch'i, the inhalation of purity and the exhalation of tension, pain or impurity.

Hold as long as is comfortable. With patient practice, increase the length of time you can hold the position.

THE PREPARATION

PART FIVE

Silently thou fliest upward in the morning.
The Book of the Seal of the Heart

THE STANCES

Correct stances are an essential part of all Wu Shu training and vital to Pa Tuan Tsin if it is to be practised correctly and to its full advantage. The way we stand, the exact position of our feet, the position of trunk, shoulders and head should be practised and perfected first. Their purpose is to strengthen the legs and lower trunk, improve balance and agility. In combat Wu Shu, this concentration of Ch'i in the lower body is channelled into amazing leaping and kicking power. Our purpose is a far gentler and more beneficial one, so let's get started on the fundamentals.

All foot and leg positions play a most important part in the exercises. Think of them as the basic steps in military drill ... standing to attention, properly at ease, right, left, about-turn and so on. Remember also that agility begins and ends with the legs. If the leg muscles are strong, sinews supple, ankle, knees and hip joints mobile, your every step becomes lighter; to walk, run or jump becomes a pleasure rather than an effort.

You may already possess a pair of sturdy legs with good thigh and calf muscles developed and maintained by regular rounds of golf, chasing a tennis ball, swimming, jogging or any other method of building leg power. If you have, you will no doubt find these stances easier to master than someone who has not. The stances may look simple and elementary to an athlete, but it is best not to under-estimate their effectiveness until you have tried them and learned to hold them steadily for the required periods of time.

Each stance is based on concentrating the strength of one leg against the other, by the shifting of body-weight with precise footwork. When practised properly, a minute or two in a particular stance can have the same result as a half-dozen turns around the block or running up and down a flight of stairs.

Correct posture is also essential. You may find it a little awkward at first, remembering to keep head, back, elbows, shoulders and stomach at the correct angles, at the same time concentrating on the positioning of your feet and legs. Your body will very soon respond and straighten to its natural points of balance much in the same way as it does when riding, dancing or swimming. The stances are all natural movements and your body will adjust and coordinate accordingly.

As there is no instructor to square a shoulder, tuck in an elbow, straighten a neck or back, pull a stomach into line, bend a knee or position a foot, you must check your own stance. Until you become naturally and comfortably accustomed to it, it is very helpful to practise in front of a full-length mirror.

Progress in the stances, once you have them right, is measured by the time for which you can hold them. In the early stages, you may find it difficult to hold a stance for more than a few seconds. This does not matter. Keep a stopwatch or clock with a second hand where you can see it. A few seconds gained each day or even each week is all you need. If you have had any previous leg, back or internal injury (such as hernia) it may be wise to show the stances to your doctor and seek approval before throwing yourself into them. After a month of practice, you will find that which was unendurable after thirty seconds is now comfortable for up to several minutes. You may find it necessary to practise the stances for the first week before beginning Pa Tuan Tsin.

Here they are, then, beginning with the foundation stance upon which all others are built and from which they are all reached, the Horse Stance.

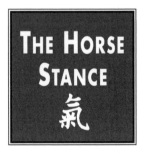

THE HORSE STANCE
氣

The Horse Stance is the rock upon which most Wu Shu forms are built. It is the stance that the old Masters had their pupils practise for up to three years before deciding if they were worth teaching further. When the Horse Stance is perfected, nothing and no one can shift it ... which is perhaps why it is also the basic fighting stance.

It is called the Horse Stance simply because the posture is that of riding an invisible horse. The feet are wide apart, the knees bent and the seat lowered into a non-existent saddle, whilst the hands grip imaginary reins in what is known as the Punch Posture.

Apart from its importance to balance, the Horse Stance begins to give immediate benefit to general health. It strengthens the legs evenly, developing reflex stability and making it less likely for you to trip, fall, be pushed or knocked down. It greatly improves circulation, aids digestion and helps constipation.

The very first step is to find the exact point of balance for your particular weight and size — which means deciding the correct distance that your feet should be apart. This is done by measuring or 'opening' the stance with your feet, as shown in Figure 1 (on page

96). Once this is discovered, the need to measure your distance can be dispensed with as practice continues. By the end of the second or third week, you will be able to open your stances comfortably and naturally, as you become familiar with your invisible horse.

With the feet properly spaced and toes pointed straight to the front, you allow the knees to bend and lower yourself into the sitting position. At first, you may find a tendency to lean forward but gradually (some faster than others), you will learn to straighten in the 'saddle' and sit back comfortably. With the stomach in, the back, head and entire upper body will be in a straight line when viewed from the side. It may take a while to achieve this erect posture and perfect it but, remember, each time you practise it the effort is doing you good.

You will also find that, no matter how athletic you are, the Horse Stance will tire you fairly quickly: your thigh muscles will ache and you will feel the urge to straighten up to relieve it. It is the willpower to ignore this urge, to persevere a little longer (always within your own limits) that develops the stance.

The ultimate question in the Horse Stance is how low you can go. The lower the stance the better its effect, but this takes time. Don't worry if at first you feel 'tall in the saddle', and don't force yourself to a point of overexertion. It is better to practise in a higher (Half-horse) position, and gradually lower a little at each session, than to subject yourself to too much strain too quickly. As your legs strengthen, you will find yourself lowering the stance easily and automatically.

Another and slightly more urgent question you will find yourself asking is 'How long am I expected to hold this position?'. Again, this is a matter of individual effort. The answer is 'As long as you can, with as much initial discomfort as you can stand without overdoing it.' There is no yardstick but your own. It is just as well to remember that no progress is possible in any form of exercise without continued effort. Perhaps it's worth mentioning that an advanced Wu Shu practitioner can hold the Horse Stance indefinitely and would think nothing of a half an hour without shifting.

If you can build up to, say, five minutes in the first few months, you will be doing very well. A clock with a second hand will tell you how you are progressing. So long as you add a few seconds each day or even each week, you are making progress. *It is better to begin with a higher but correct stance for longer periods than a lower, incorrect stance for short exhausting bouts.*

When the stance is perfected, it forces Ch'i down to the lower abdomen and is distributed between the spread legs to the feet. It makes for perfect stability, ease of balance and a lightness of movement you will never have experienced in normal motion.

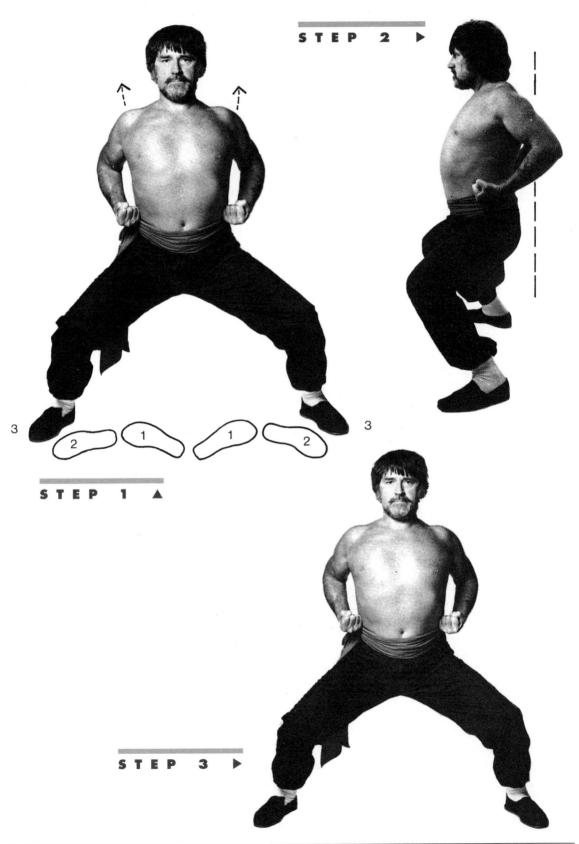

STEP 2 ▶

3

2 1 1 2

STEP 1 ▲

STEP 3 ▶

The Bow Stance is so called because the widespread feet and stretched legs, one straight as an arrow, the other bent and the body curved, could be seen as a fully drawn bow, its shaft poised for flight. This is not an exaggerated interpretation. The Bow Stance, when applied to the fighting technique, is used to launch an attack, the rear leg firing the strike deep into the opponent's defences.

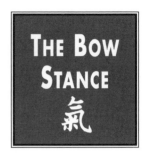

Its purpose for us is far less aggressive. The Bow Stance is designed to further promote solid balance and strengthen both legs. As a variation of the Horse Stance, it eventually leads to the 'rooting' of Ch'i, making it almost impossible to lose balance.

Until you become accustomed to opening the Bow Stance accurately and comfortably it is best reached through the Horse Stance:

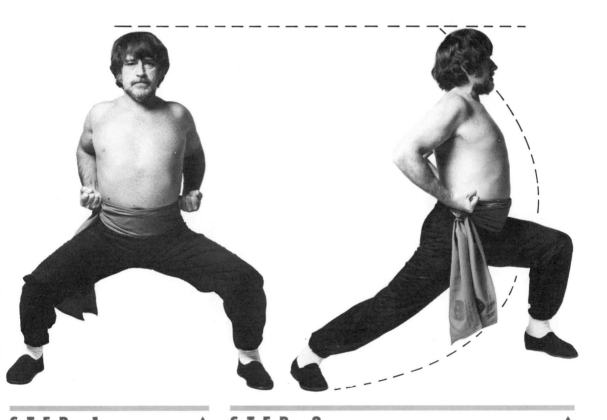

S T E P   1   ▲

Open your Horse Stance.

S T E P   2   ▲

Pivot to the left on the soles of the feet until the right leg is straight at the knee, toe pointing to 11 o'clock. The left leg is bent as far forward as possible, toe in line with the knee. The trunk is upright from the waist, arms and shoulders drawn back hard (but relaxed). Eighty per cent of the body-weight is thrown forward on to the bent left leg. Hold the stance for as long as possible. When the weight on the left leg becomes excessive, pivot back to the Horse Stance without raising the head level or rising on the knees.

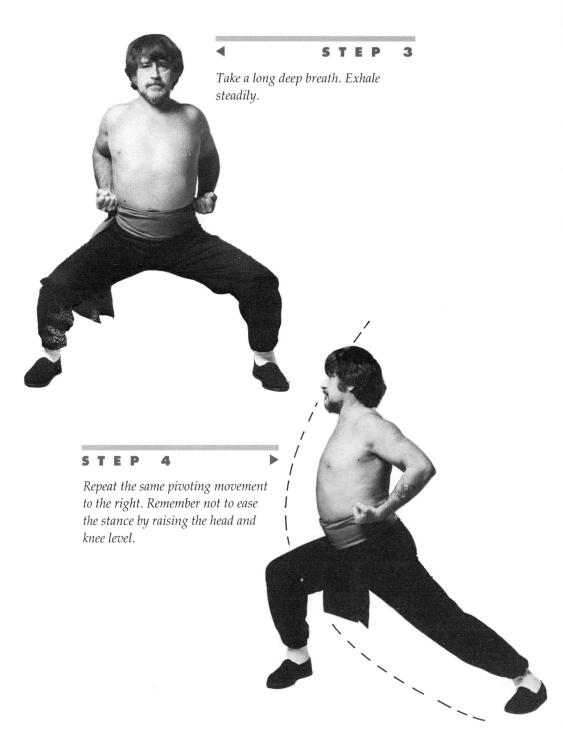

STEP 3

Take a long deep breath. Exhale steadily.

STEP 4

Repeat the same pivoting movement to the right. Remember not to ease the stance by raising the head and knee level.

At first, you may find moving from Horse to Right Bow, to Horse, to Left Bow without rising too difficult. If so, don't worry, settle into each stance in the way most comfortable to you until you are able to complete all three movements without rising. Hold the stance for a minute or two, extending your time as best you can.

The Seven Star Stance is considered the classic fighting stance of the Northern Shaolin school of the Praying Mantis. It is an attack stance from which the 'short hand' close-range engagement is launched, the right heel often used as a strike against an opponent's instep or a scoop to unbalance him/her. Our less formidable purpose is to further perfect balance and strengthen leg work.

The Seven Star is also opened from the Horse Stance.

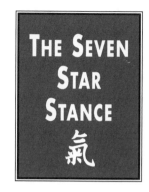

THE SEVEN STAR STANCE
氣

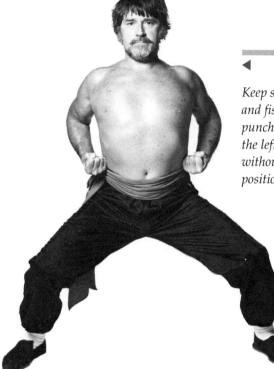

◀ **STEP 1**

Keep shoulders, elbows and fists tucked into the punch posture. Leave the left foot where it is without shifting its position.

STEP 2 ▶

Lean 80 per cent of the body-weight on to the left leg, bending it accordingly. Stretch the right leg, rigid and locked at the knee, resting lightly on the heel of the foot. Upper body twists to face the right in line with the upraised toe. When the stance is correct, most of the body-weight will be taken up on the half-bent left leg. The right heel will be lightly resting on the floor.

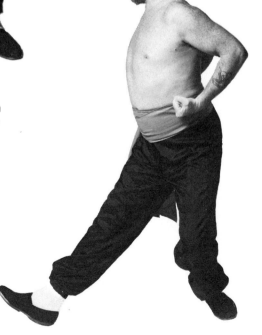

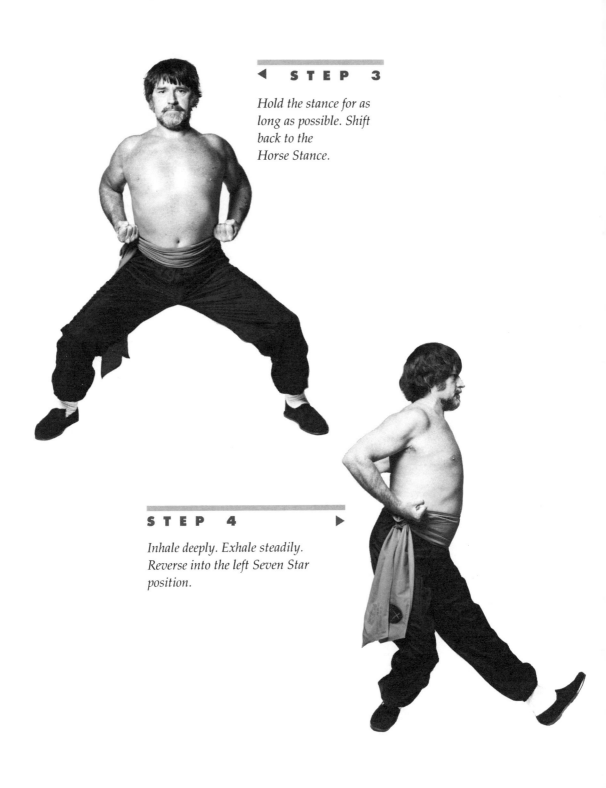

◄ **STEP 3**

Hold the stance for as long as possible. Shift back to the Horse Stance.

STEP 4 ►

Inhale deeply. Exhale steadily. Reverse into the left Seven Star position.

You must expect to find this stance quite difficult to maintain for any length of time because of strain on the bent leg. Be patient and gradually increase the seconds as the legs become stronger.

The Half-knee Stance is a variation of the Seven Star. It is simply a feinting manoeuvre intended to give the opponent the impression of retreat while remaining poised to spring from the bent back leg.

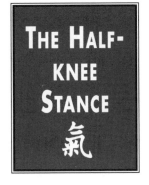

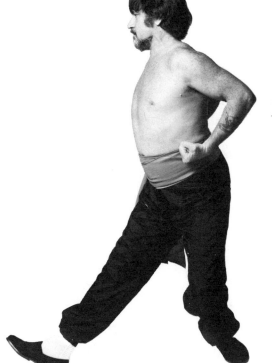

◄ **S T E P   1**

The Seven Star Stance is adopted.

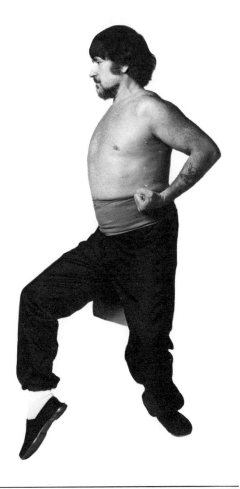

S T E P   2 ▶

The right leg is drawn back until the knee is half bent and the toe rests very lightly on the floor. Again, most of the body-weight is taken by the 'springing' leg.

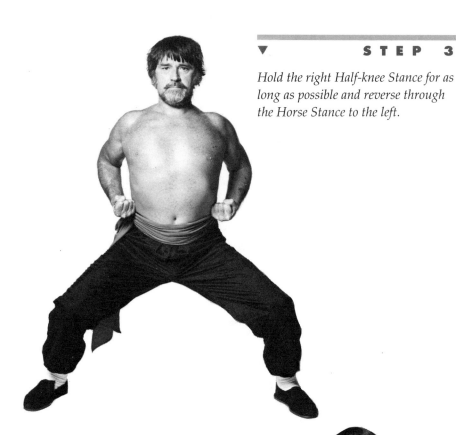

Hold the right Half-knee Stance for as long as possible and reverse through the Horse Stance to the left.

The same degree of strain will again be placed on the prop, or spring, leg. The outstretched toe should be so lightly poised as to pass a sheet of paper beneath it. At first this toe (pointed in much the same way as a ballet dancer) may rely on too much pressure against the floor; this will ease as the spring leg learns to take more and more weight and balance upon itself. Think of it as a tightrope walker feeling for the next step.

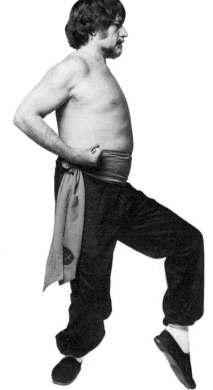

The Front Cross Stance is an evasive tactic that develops great agility. It is essentially another leg and balance exercise which, although not utilised in Pa Tuan Tsin, is a very worthwhile part of your program. Aimed at an opponent attacking from the side, it advances swiftly under the attacking guard and offers a low strike.

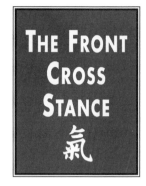

THE FRONT CROSS STANCE
氣

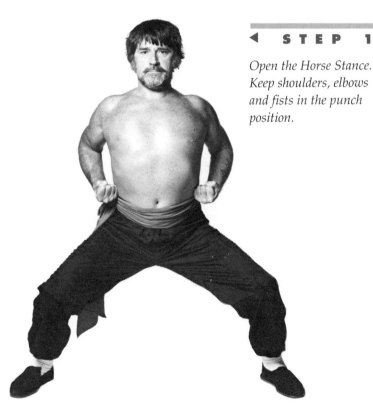

◄ **STEP 1**

Open the Horse Stance. Keep shoulders, elbows and fists in the punch position.

STEP 2 ►

Bring the left leg across the right knee and sink into a crouch. Left foot flat on the floor, toe at 9 o'clock, right heel raised, toe at 11 o'clock. Body-weight is evenly distributed on both legs. Hold as long as possible.

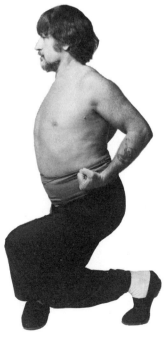

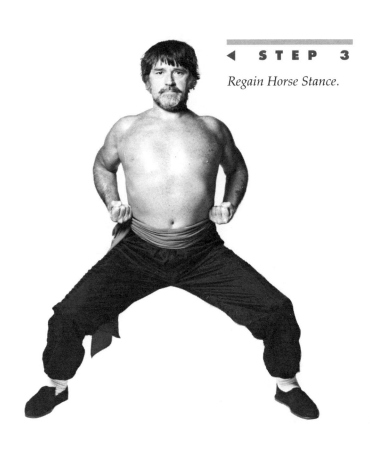

Regain Horse Stance.

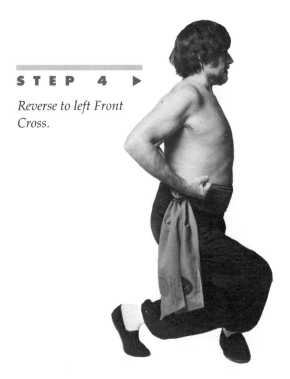

S T E P 4 ▶

Reverse to left Front Cross.

The Back Cross Stance is a similar evasive tactic, this time defending to the front with the same effect.

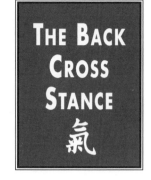

◄ **STEP 1**

Open the Horse Stance and punch position.

STEP 2 ►

Cross the left leg behind the right, left heel raised, toe at 12 o'clock. Right heel flat, toe at 11 o'clock. Sink into a crouch position. Upper body facing front.

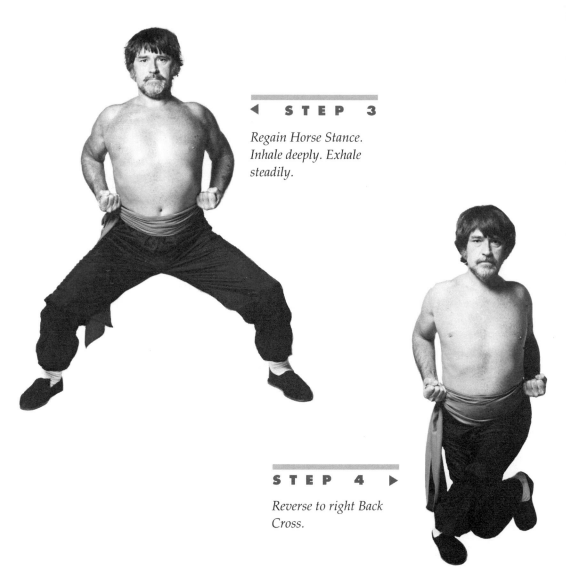

◀ **S T E P   3**

Regain Horse Stance.
Inhale deeply. Exhale
steadily.

S T E P   4 ▶

Reverse to right Back
Cross.

Both of these exercises are particularly hard on the legs at first, and you may find it difficult to retain balance. After a few weeks of practice, however, you will be able to slip from one to the other without rising.

Once the stances are understood and you find you can open them quite easily, you can progress to the warm-up exercises.

THE WARM-UP EXERCISES

The warm-up exercises are really the limbering-up process before the practice of Wu Shu proper. They are a prelude to the Chien Taos, which are dance-like movements performed in continual sequence. They will become second nature before being applied to actual sparring sessions. It is much as a ballet dancer will go through a stretching routine on the bar before a performance, or a boxer will warm up on the speed ball before a fight. As such, the warm-up is not essential. You can perform Pa Tuan Tsin without it. It is, however, a highly effective way of getting your circulation going, taking out any kinks in your body and preparing your mind for concentration.

The warm-up is a sinew-stretching and muscle-loosening procedure designed to minimise strain, starting with the head and neck, arms and shoulders, waist and abdomen, legs and feet. The full set of eight warm-up exercises each repeated eight times will take no more than fifteen extra minutes and is well worth making time for if you can.

In the beginning, the warm-up exercises should be approached carefully and without impatience. Remember, you are testing yourself joint by joint, sinew by sinew, muscle by muscle. Even if you are fit and accustomed to regular exercise, there may well be effort involved with which your body is not familiar. A pulled muscle or sprained sinew is not only a very painful way of interrupting your progress but, without the advice and encouragement of an instructor, it can easily dampen your enthusiasm to continue.

Bear in mind that, no matter how receptive or flexible your attitude may be, however firm your resolution, there will be times in the first few weeks when you will be sorely tempted to drop out. The only way to guard against such temptation is to persevere. Approach each exercise slowly and without force, even gingerly at first. Be satisfied with a little progress each day (or week). Do not push yourself too soon: your body will make its own demands and decisions. If you can complete the first month, even on alternate days, you will be sufficiently convinced to continue.

The only rule, if you decide to wisely include the warm-up in your routine, is not to rest or sit down between exercises. Complete each set of repetitions as instructed, take one long deep breath, count to six, exhale slowly and continue with the next set without leaving your position. When the warm-up is finished, relax for a few moments, but keep your circulation going by walking about the room or garden. *Do not sit or lie down.* Refresh yourself with water or green tea.

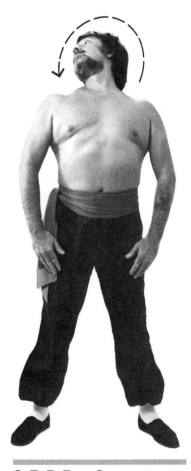

HEAD ROLLING
氣

Relax. Stand with feet together, hands loosely at sides.

You may experience considerable creakings and crackings, particularly when rolling the head back over the spine, which may pop like the pulling of a knuckle joint. It simply shows that your neck is in need of exercise and will diminish with practice.

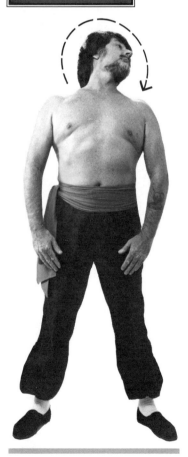
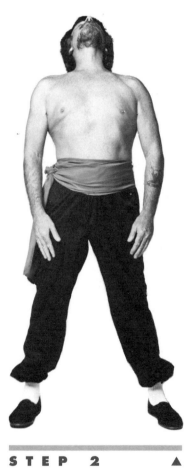

S T E P   2 ▲

Make sure to stretch the neck as far forward, to the side and back as possible. Complete three circles and return Chin to chest.

S T E P   1 ▲

Roll the head slowly to the left in a clockwise direction.

S T E P   3 ▲

Repeat three times to the right.

Relax. Stand with feet apart, hands loosely at sides.

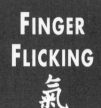

FINGER FLICKING

氣

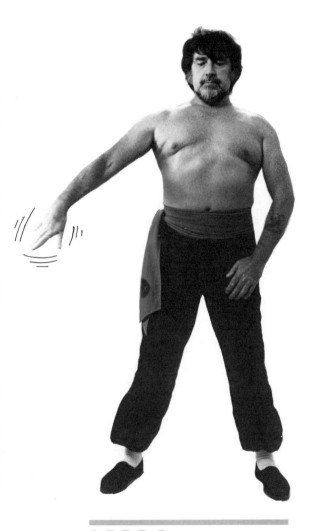

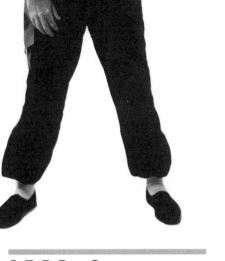

STEP 1 ▲

Move the right hand about 30 centimetres away from your body and commence to flick vigorously the loose fingers as though trying to rid them of something sticky or to shake off drops of water. Continue for about 10 seconds or until the whole hand is tingling with circulation.

STEP 2 ▲

Return right hand to the side and repeat with the left hand.

INHALE SLOWLY AND DEEPLY.
HOLD FOR SILENT COUNT OF SIX.
EXHALE SLOWLY AND STEADILY.

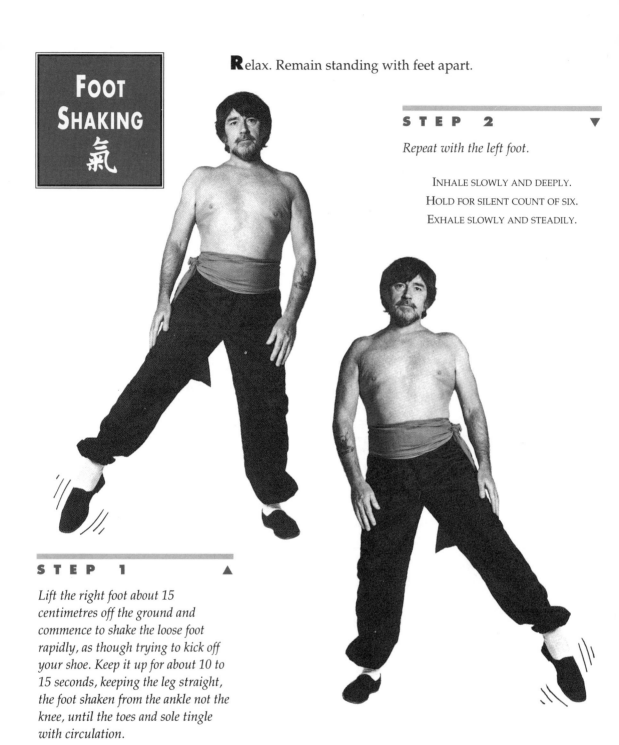

FOOT SHAKING

氣

Relax. Remain standing with feet apart.

STEP 2 ▼

Repeat with the left foot.

INHALE SLOWLY AND DEEPLY.
HOLD FOR SILENT COUNT OF SIX.
EXHALE SLOWLY AND STEADILY.

STEP 1 ▲

Lift the right foot about 15 centimetres off the ground and commence to shake the loose foot rapidly, as though trying to kick off your shoe. Keep it up for about 10 to 15 seconds, keeping the leg straight, the foot shaken from the ankle not the knee, until the toes and sole tingle with circulation.

The momentary pulsing you will experience in the palms and fingers, soles and toes is caused by a forced quickening of the blood. When shaking the foot, you may tend to lose balance. Stop and try again: you will very soon learn to retain it. The purpose of this simple opening exercise is to stimulate circulation, loosen muscles and stretch sinews, and also to relax you.

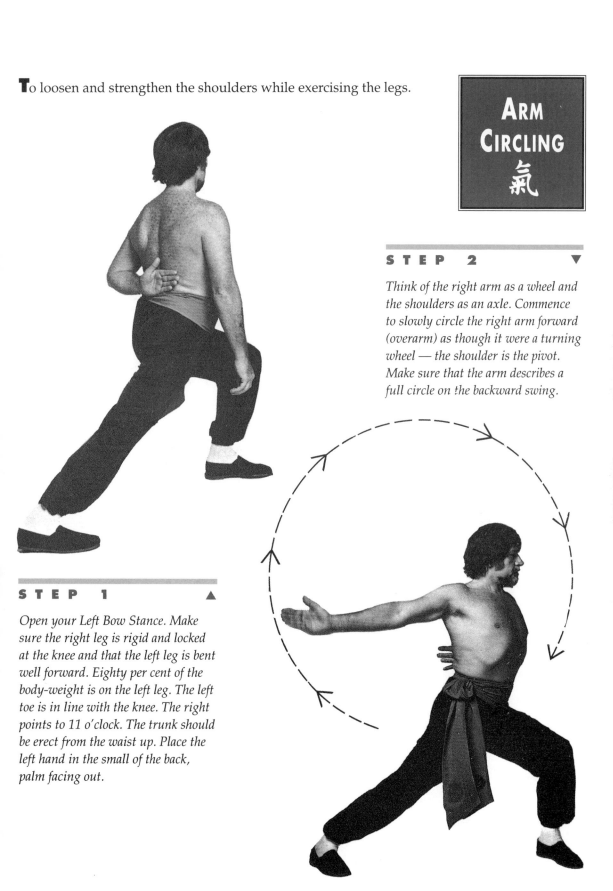

To loosen and strengthen the shoulders while exercising the legs.

ARM CIRCLING
氣

STEP 2 ▼

Think of the right arm as a wheel and the shoulders as an axle. Commence to slowly circle the right arm forward (overarm) as though it were a turning wheel — the shoulder is the pivot. Make sure that the arm describes a full circle on the backward swing.

STEP 1 ▲

Open your Left Bow Stance. Make sure the right leg is rigid and locked at the knee and that the left leg is bent well forward. Eighty per cent of the body-weight is on the left leg. The left toe is in line with the knee. The right points to 11 o'clock. The trunk should be erect from the waist up. Place the left hand in the small of the back, palm facing out.

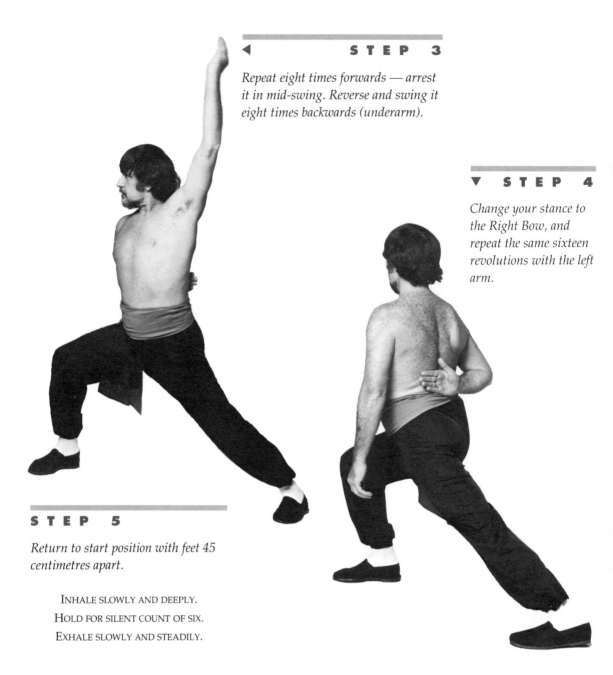

◄ STEP 3

Repeat eight times forwards — arrest it in mid-swing. Reverse and swing it eight times backwards (underarm).

▼ STEP 4

Change your stance to the Right Bow, and repeat the same sixteen revolutions with the left arm.

STEP 5

Return to start position with feet 45 centimetres apart.

INHALE SLOWLY AND DEEPLY.
HOLD FOR SILENT COUNT OF SIX.
EXHALE SLOWLY AND STEADILY.

Depending on the suppleness of your shoulders, you may experience a degree of popping and 'grinding' in the circling shoulder joint — plus a tendency for the circling arm to veer to the side on the backward swing as though the wheel revolved on a buckled axle. Don't straighten it by force, bend it gently to your will with patience, a little more each day until it is as easily turned backwards as it is forwards. The cracking of the shoulder ligament is to be expected if the joint is at all stiff. It will soon disappear as the shoulder becomes supple.

To strengthen the abdominal area and reduce the waistline while exercising the spine and back muscles. Relax.

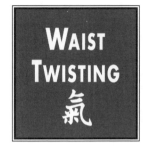

WAIST TWISTING
氣

STEP 1

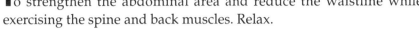

Still standing with feet apart, raise the right hand above the head, palm uppermost, hand bent to a right angle from the wrist, fingers pointing left. Lower the left hand behind the back, palm down, hand bent at a right angle to the wrist, fingers pointing right.

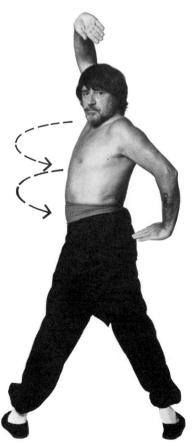

STEP 2

Lock legs and hips to the front. Relax the trunk from the waist up. Commence twisting the upper body to the left and look behind you as far as possible. Repeat sixteen times.

INHALE SLOWLY AND DEEPLY.

HOLD FOR SILENT COUNT OF SIX.

EXHALE SLOWLY AND STEADILY.

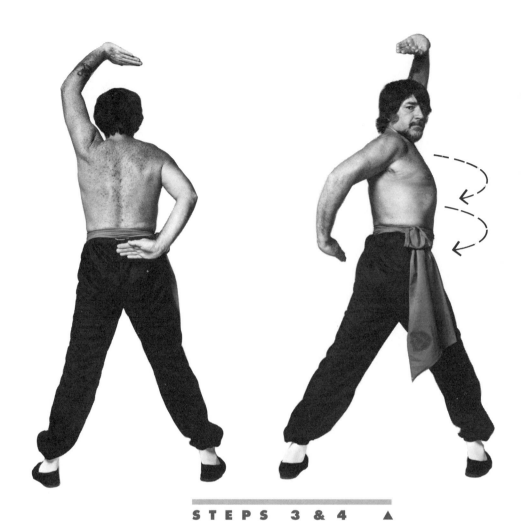

STEPS 3 & 4 ▲

*Reverse hands and repeat sixteen
times to the right.*

INHALE SLOWLY AND DEEPLY.
HOLD FOR SILENT COUNT OF SIX.
EXHALE SLOWLY AND STEADILY.

At first, you will find a tendency to swing the hips: the pivot must be
from the waist, not the hips. Concentrate on keeping the feet in
position and the legs and hips locked to the front, not on how far you
can turn. Waist twisting flexibility will quickly increase with practice.

To exercise the kidney region and stomach muscles. Relax.

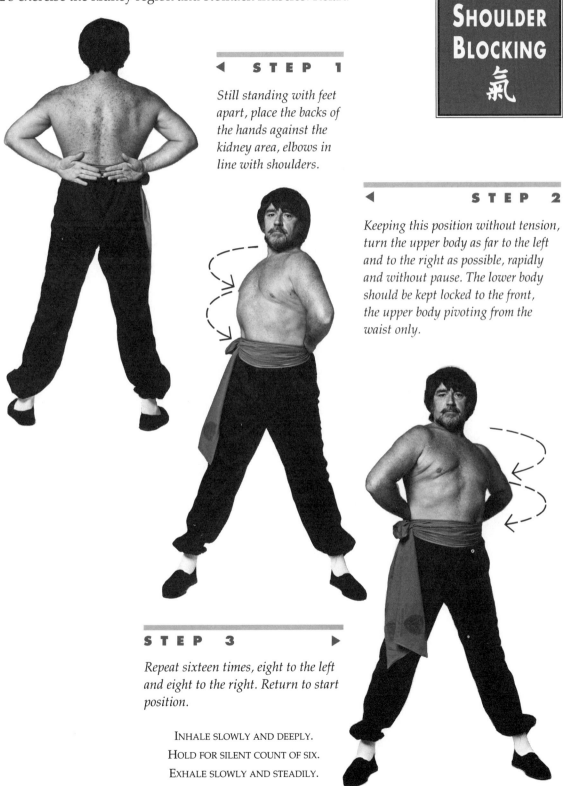

◀ **S T E P   1**

Still standing with feet apart, place the backs of the hands against the kidney area, elbows in line with shoulders.

◀ **S T E P   2**

Keeping this position without tension, turn the upper body as far to the left and to the right as possible, rapidly and without pause. The lower body should be kept locked to the front, the upper body pivoting from the waist only.

S T E P   3 ▶

Repeat sixteen times, eight to the left and eight to the right. Return to start position.

INHALE SLOWLY AND DEEPLY.
HOLD FOR SILENT COUNT OF SIX.
EXHALE SLOWLY AND STEADILY.

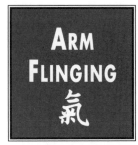

ARM FLINGING
氣

To loosen and strengthen shoulders and arms, whilst exercising the chest. Relax.

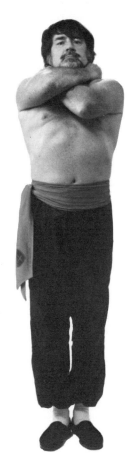

◄ STEP 1

Draw the feet together until they are touching. Cross the forearms (left over right) under the Chin with fists loosely closed.

◄ STEP 2

Fling arms wide, outward and back with as much force as you can muster. Make sure the outflung arms remain at shoulder level, no higher and no lower. As the arms travel backwards, tighten your fists so that they are fully tensed at the end of the fling. Think of them as weights used to gain that extra centimetre to the rear. Relax the fists and arms as they return to the chest and repeat sixteen times.

INHALE SLOWLY
AND DEEPLY.

HOLD FOR SILENT COUNT
OF SIX.

EXHALE SLOWLY
AND STEADILY.

You may find a tendency to lean either forwards or backwards with the momentum of arm flinging, also to lower the arms on the backward swing. Concentrate on remaining erect and on reaching as far to the rear as possible without lowering the arms. Go gently at first, increase the power as you feel the need.

To exercise the back and stretch leg sinews and to increase general flexibility. Relax.

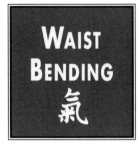

STEP 2 ▼

Raise the hands above the head and bring them down to touch the ground as far to the left as possible. Without fully straightening, repeat eight times, each time trying to reach a little further and lower to the left.

STEP 1 ▲

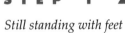

Still standing with feet 45 centimetres apart, open them about another 30 centimetres.

STEP 3 ▲

Straighten with hands above the head and repeat eight times to the right. Straighten to start position.

INHALE SLOWLY AND DEEPLY.
HOLD FOR SILENT COUNT OF SIX.
EXHALE SLOWLY AND STEADILY.

SEVEN STAR, CHIN-TO-TOE

氣

To stretch and exercise legs, back and stomach. To increase flexibility. Relax.

STEP 1 ▶

Take up the left Seven Star Stance. Hands on hips. Bend forward along the outstretched leg as far as you can, aiming the point of the Chin at the raised toe. Half rise and repeat sixteen times.

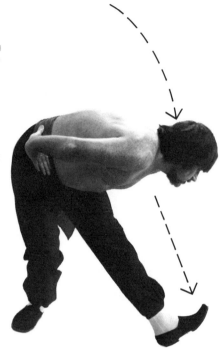

STEP 2 ▶

Reverse to the right Seven Star and repeat sixteen times. Straighten to start position.

INHALE SLOWLY AND DEEPLY.
HOLD FOR SILENT COUNT OF SIX.
EXHALE SLOWLY AND STEADILY.

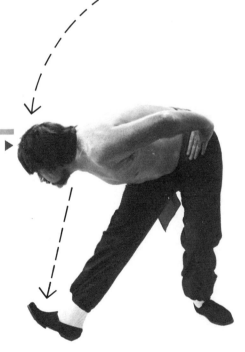

To stretch and strengthen legs and spine. To increase flexibility. This simple variation of Seven Star uses the foot for leverage to increase the effectiveness. Depending on your waistline, you may find a considerable distance between your nose and your knee, a gap that will close surprisingly quickly with regular practice.

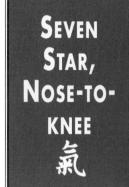
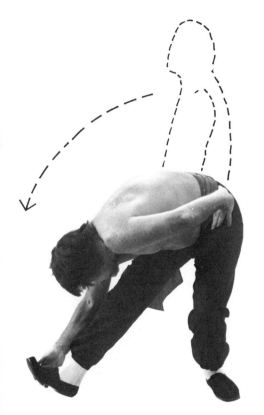

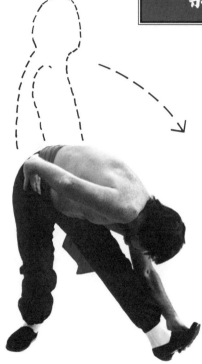

CAUTION Approach all such forward bending exercises very carefully if you have any back problems.

ANKLE ROTATING

氣

To loosen and strengthen the ankles. Relax.

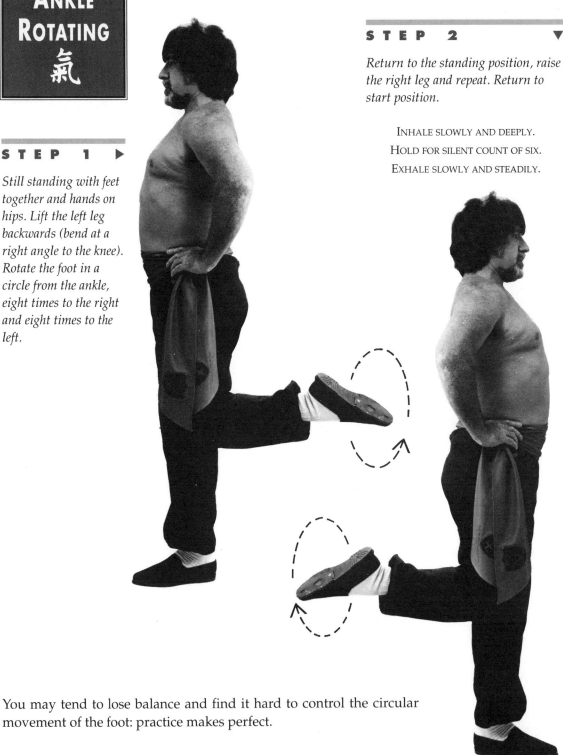

STEP 1 ▶

Still standing with feet together and hands on hips. Lift the left leg backwards (bend at a right angle to the knee). Rotate the foot in a circle from the ankle, eight times to the right and eight times to the left.

STEP 2 ▼

Return to the standing position, raise the right leg and repeat. Return to start position.

INHALE SLOWLY AND DEEPLY.
HOLD FOR SILENT COUNT OF SIX.
EXHALE SLOWLY AND STEADILY.

You may tend to lose balance and find it hard to control the circular movement of the foot: practice makes perfect.

This exercise for agility may seem awkward at first but it is excellent for loosening and strengthening the knees.

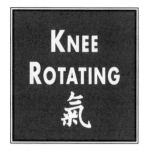

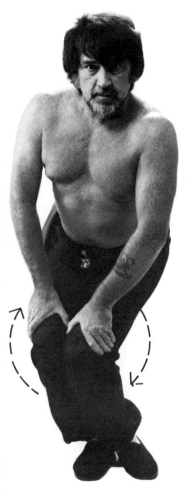

◄ **S T E P 1**

Stand with feet and legs close together. Bend the knees until you can grip each leg just above the knee, while keeping the arms straight. Using that position as a pivot, describe a deep circle around it; eight times to the right.

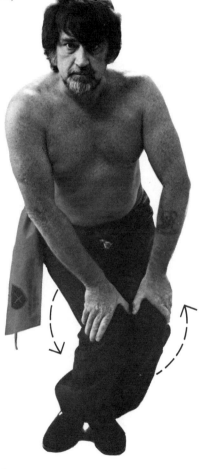

S T E P 2 ►

Without pausing or straightening the legs, repeat eight times to the left.

INHALE SLOWLY AND DEEPLY.

HOLD FOR SILENT COUNT OF SIX.

EXHALE SLOWLY AND STEADILY.

You have now completed the warm-up exercises in as little as ten minutes, allowing for thirty-second breath pauses. You have loosened the neck, arm and leg muscles, got your circulation going, worked down to shoulders, arms, waist, knees and ankles. Even if time does not permit these exercises to be carried out every day, working through them every other day or even three times a week will give you a very nice feeling of relaxed lightness while toning you up, strengthening and loosening taut joints and sinews. This is a marvellous prelude to Pa Tuan Tsin.

THE VITAL KNEECAP

Many Kung Fu training methods were devised a very long time ago — long before anyone had heard of sports medicine — if you hurt yourself in training, you healed yourself, endured or dropped out. Even modern martial arts still base many of their fundamental exercises on those laid down centuries ago by an entirely different breed of people living under entirely different conditions who, whilst possessing an intricate knowledge of the human anatomy, were not quite as concerned about the prospect of sports injury and foot placement as we are today. Enlightened schools have modified some aspects of their training program to better suit the genetic changes that have occurred since the basic stances were first created more than 2000 years ago.

One of the modifications concerns us here. It is the position of the foot when forming the Bow Stance. The time-honoured way was to keep the foot of the bent leg in the Horse Stance position — that is to say — pivot on the ball of the foot of the straight outstretched leg but throw all body-weight upon the bent knee, leaving the foot at right angles to it. Knee specialists in sports injury clinics have learned that this could damage or at least overstretch the cruciate ligaments, causing a misalignment of the patella (kneecap) when the knee can suddenly 'give' under stress (as in running, going downhill, or trying to squat). Unlike muscles, ligaments do not contract or tighten up again, and that is why these knee injuries, which eventually weaken knees, are such a nuisance to athletes. Once weakened in this way they are far more difficult to treat.

Note: The forward foot can be angled half-way between Steps 1 and 2.

The modification recommended by sports medicine experts is to keep the knee in line with the foot (knee over toe) so that the pressure of body-weight is shared by the foot and not left entirely to the knee. This is particularly important in training where the Bow Stance is consistently used or in Chi Kung exercises where the Bow Stance is held for long periods.

Pa Tuan Tsin – Eight Precious Sets of Exercises

The mountain air is beautiful in the sunset.
I drink of it as from a snow-fed stream.
It purifies me, it strengthens me, it calms me.

Tao

PART
SIX

We are now ready to begin Pa Tuan Tsin. You have chosen the spot in which you feel most natural and where the air is at its best; you are dressed in loose-fitting, comfortable clothing with ample leg room, your footwear is light and flat-bottomed, the sash around your waist is soft and not tied too tightly. You are stripped of metal accessories, you have eaten nothing for at least two hours and taken no alcohol for at least six. There is a pitcher of cool to warm boiled water or hot green tea nearby in case you need it. You remember that all inhalation and exhalation must always be through the nose, never through the mouth (unless exhalation is so instructed). All breathing should be concentrated on the slow, silent and deep. The words *patience*, *discipline*, *fortitude* and *faith* are firmly in mind.

SCOOP THE STREAM

氣

The first exercise is one of the simplest and most pleasant to perform. It is so named because the second movement gives the impression of scooping water from a stream and drinking from the cupped hands.

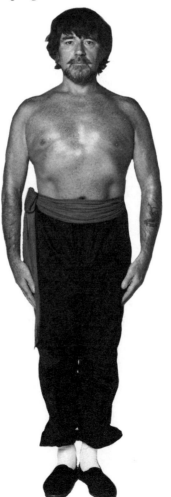

THE BENEFIT It is excellent for expanding the lungs and stretching the ribcage. It also circulates the dormant Ch'i from the lower abdomen to the top of the spinal column and to the forehead. It gives you a general lift and generates immediate alertness. A good way to wake up and get started.

◄ **STEP 1**

Relax. Take up your position, standing with feet together and hands loosely at sides, fix your eyes on a chosen object.

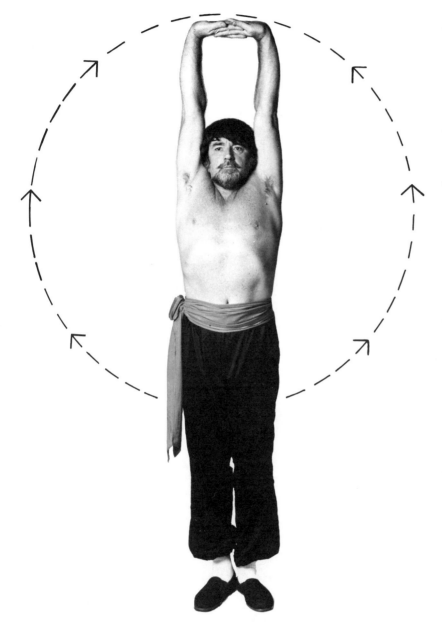

Empty the lungs. Inhale as slowly as you can while raising the hands (palms down) until the fingertips touch above the head (palms now up). The time required for the movement should coincide with the length of your breath. Stretch the body upward to its fullest extent without raising the heels. Imagine that you are supporting a great weight with your two palms. Hold for the silent count of three. Exhale slowly and steadily while reversing the movement and lowering the hands in time with the exhalation until they are gently back at your sides and the lungs are drained of air. Pause for the silent count of three.

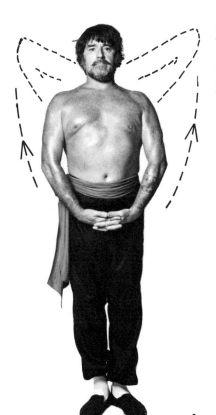

◄ **STEP 3**

Intertwine the fingers,
forming a scoop, palms
uppermost. Inhale
slowly and deeply while
raising 'the scoop'
to the lips, bent arms
in line with shoulders,
elbows raised as high
as possible.

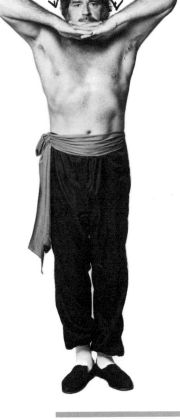

STEP 4 ▲

To the silent count of
three, turn the scoop
over (palms down)
and exhale steadily
while reversing the
movement.

STEP 5 ▶

Stretch the arms downward to their
fullest extent as though pressing the
palms down on a spring-loaded
weight. Hold for the silent count of
three. Return the relaxed hands to the
sides and repeat both movements
eight times.

The second exercise is so-called because of its ultimate stretching power. The uppermost hand and flattened palm really seem to be supporting the sky.

THE BENEFIT A variation of Scoop the Stream, in which the active points are the liver and the shoulders. Ch'i is circulated from the liver to the shoulders alternately, conditioning the liver, stimulating its function while relieving the shoulders of strain, and stretching the entire body to its fullest extent.

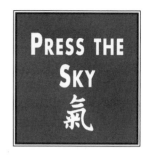

PRESS THE SKY
氣

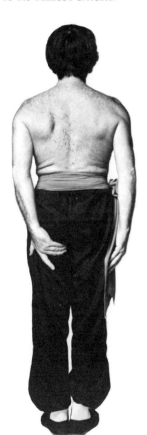

◀ STEP 1

Relax. Remain in position with feet together.

Reach behind with the left hand and firmly clasp the back of the thigh, just below the left buttock.

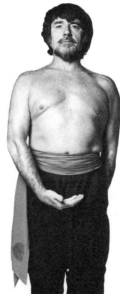

◀ STEP 2

Drain the lungs of air. Form a 'cup' with the right hand hooked at the wrist.

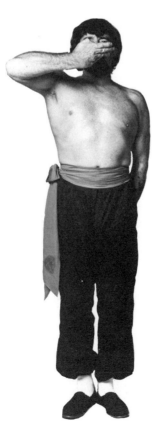

◀ STEP 3

Inhale slowly and deeply while raising the cup to the lips, elbow in line with shoulder.

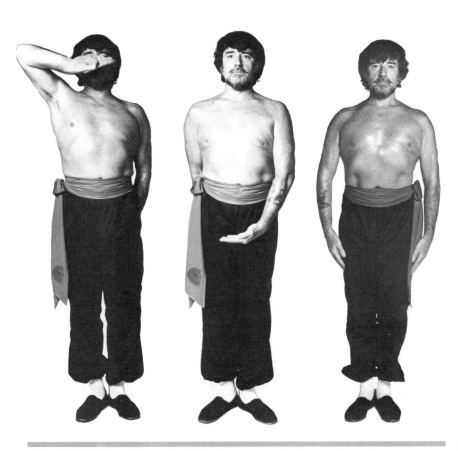

*Without pause, turn the cup outward
and over, rise on your toes and
continue inhaling until the right arm
is 'pressing the sky'. From toes to
upturned palm, your body is stretched
to its absolute utmost and full of air.
Hold for the count of three.*

STEPS 5, 6 & 7 ▲

*Exhale slowly and steadily and reverse the action exactly: lower the upturned
palm to the lips while lowering the heels. Form the cup at the lips, lower to the
groin, relax with both hands at the sides. Reach behind with the right hand to
grasp the right back thigh below the buttock. Repeat the movements exactly with
the left hand. Complete four times with each arm.*

The third and much-revered exercise is perhaps the most 'beautiful jewel in the crown of the Precious Eight' ... at least that is how it was once described by a Shaolin priest. Its quite classical performance is reminiscent of a Chinese opera, where all sets, props and even weapons are imaginary. It is best described as the drawing of a longbow hewn from the oldest yew or blackwood, or forged of the finest steel. It is a bow that takes the strength, artistry and skill of the true archer to bend.

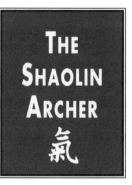

THE SHAOLIN ARCHER

THE BENEFIT This exercise can be used alone when time does not permit the full sequence, it being considered the most beneficial of the set. Its primary purpose, because of its separate (left and right) stretching, is to exercise alternate lung power. At the same time its twisting motion under pressure relieves and strengthens the liver. Executed from the Half-horse (or full Horse, if you feel like it), it also brings into play the leg, hip and spinal exercise explained under Horse Stance, plus the stretching and strengthening of sinew and joint in the arm, developing unexpected power.

Relax. Drop into a Half-horse Stance (high-seated, knees half-bent). Settle comfortably, checking your stance for perfect balance; move your foot a centimetre or two to find it.

STEP 1 ▶

Take a long, silent breath while raising the right arm and holding it at shoulder level. The left hand is on the left thigh. The right hand is relaxed from the wrist, the right arm firm but not tensed. Keep your eyes, half-closed, upon the outstretched hand. Think of nothing else but the hand. It is a beautiful thing. It is your hand, it has accompanied you and obeyed you throughout your life. It has many times saved you, it is your closest friend, without it you are lost. Love your precious hand as it moves to your will.

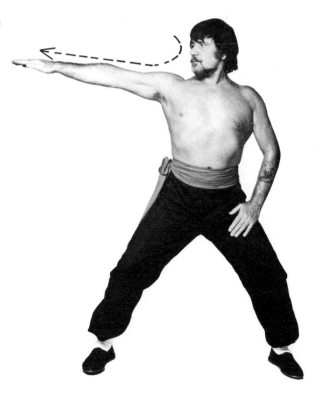

Swing the hand in its gentle state slowly across your body just below eye-level, keeping the arm locked but relaxed. Watch its progress as though it were a bird in flight, until it is across your chest and pointing left. During this flight, you are gently exhaling, emptying your lungs quietly but completely.

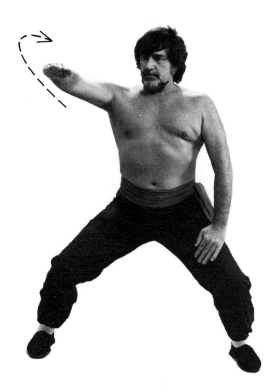

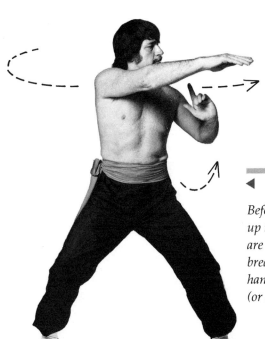

◀ STEP 3

Before it has finished travelling, bring up the bow (left hand). Your lungs are now empty and ready to draw breath. Raise the forefinger of the left hand as though its tip were a target (or a gun sight).

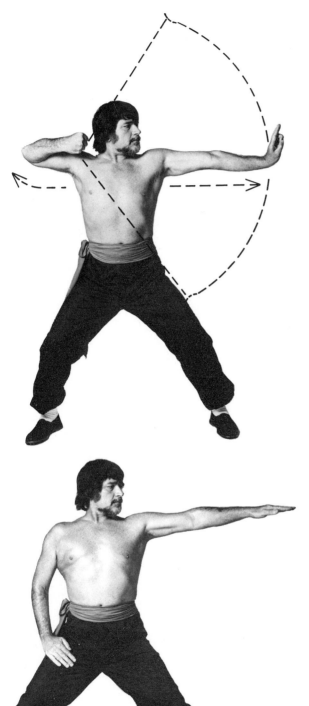

Inhale slowly, quietly, steadily, as you push out the bow to full arm's length, keeping your eyes fixed on the raised fingertip. Straighten the left arm to its fullest extent, locking the elbow until the full breath has been drawn. At the same time, the 'arrow hand' has been slowly drawn back to its fullest extent. All motion should cease with the peak of your inhalation. In other words, your movements last as long as your slowest inhalation and exhalation.

Hold the pose for the silent count of three. During that period of three seconds, with lungs fully extended, concentrate through willpower your entire bodily strength into your raised fingertip. Stretch that extended right arm to its absolute maximum and a little bit more. The elbow and wrist should tighten like a stretched rope, just the way a cat puts every ounce of power into the awakening stretch of its forelegs.

On three, begin to gently exhale and repeat the exact procedure in reverse, lowering the right hand slowly to the thigh and now relaxing the taut left hand at the wrist.

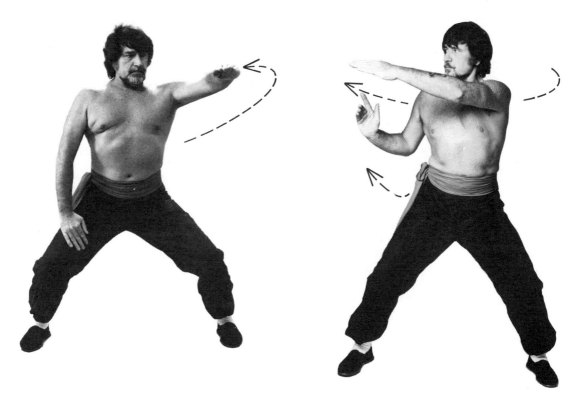

STEPS 6, 7 & 8

The left hand has now become the arrow hand and the right will raise the bow. Exhale as the left hand swings slowly into position and draw the bow to the right.

This may sound complicated but you will find that it is not. Just imagine the fitting, drawing and releasing of an imaginary bow, drawn first to the right and then to the left. Repeat four times on either side.

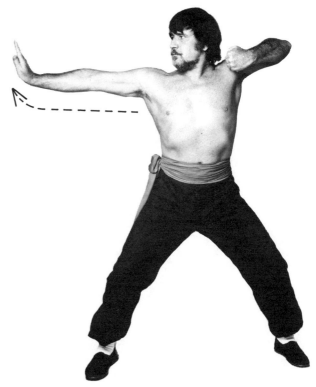

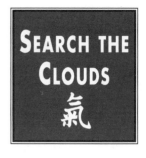
The fourth exercise is referred to in Wu Shu circles as 'a very essential health dose'. This may be an added incentive to practise it correctly as it appears quite awkward to perform and calls for considerable physical application. It is called Search the Clouds because the movements command attention upwards.

THE BENEFIT Its benefit can be seen after internal injuries such as bruises or contusion caused from heavy sparring or actual combat. This indicates its internal effectiveness. It is also accepted as a pick-up for fatigue and overexertion 'especially after sexual intimacy'. Sexual exhaustion or tiredness can interfere with bodily functions, in particular the digestive system. Searching the clouds hardly seems a recuperative procedure for a bruised or weary body, but with careful and regular practice you will find that it is.

Relax. Remain in the Half-horse Stance (or rest your legs for a moment if you must), then lower into the full Horse Stance.

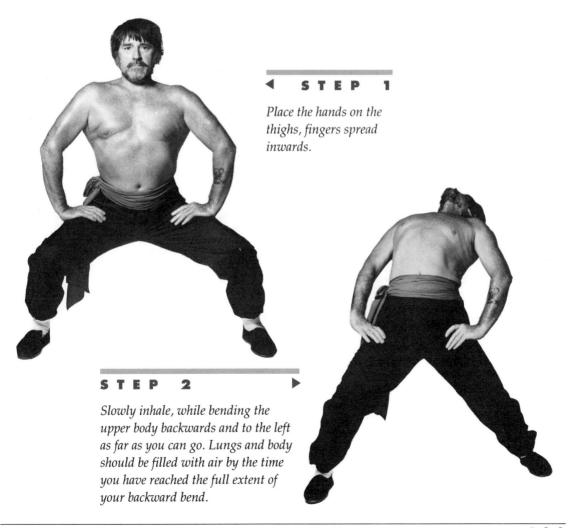

◀ **S T E P   1**

Place the hands on the thighs, fingers spread inwards.

S T E P   2 ▶

Slowly inhale, while bending the upper body backwards and to the left as far as you can go. Lungs and body should be filled with air by the time you have reached the full extent of your backward bend.

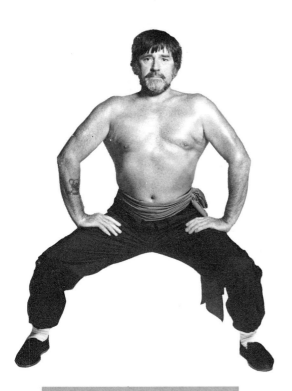

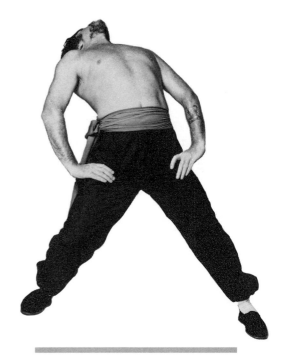

STEP 3 ▲

Hold for the silent count of three, pressing back to gain another centimetre. Exhale steadily as you bring the upper body forward to its central position, by which time the lungs and body are drained of air.

Relax. Hold for the silent count of three.

STEP 4 ▲

Repeat the movement to the right. Complete four times on each side. Close the Horse Stance and stand erect.

The fifth exercise is a combination of exercises one and two: scooping and pressing. The basic movement is that of taking the weight of a rock or nearby object in the hands, lifting it to the Chin and raising it as high above the head as possible.

THE BENEFIT It offers all-round internal benefits while bringing about the utmost in upward stretching. We have all observed the animal stretching habits, particularly feline, upon waking or rising. No authority on physical energy control and bodily relaxation could deny that stretching has considerable restorative effects.

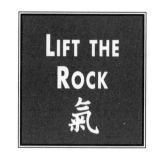

LIFT THE ROCK

氣

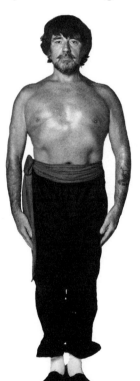

◄ **S T E P 1**

*Relax. Stand erect with feet together.
Empty the lungs of air.*

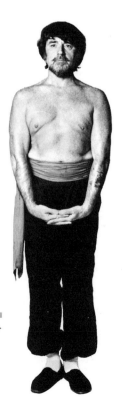

S T E P 2 ▶

*Entwine the fingers,
palms uppermost (to
accept the rock).*

S T E P 3 ▲

*Inhale slowly and deeply while
raising the joined hands level
with the Chin.*

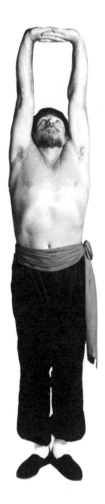

◄ **S T E P 4**

Palms outwards and upwards as you continue to press above the head. Follow the movement of your hands with your eyes until your flat, upturned palms have reached their utmost height. Strain to gain an extra fraction, to the silent count of three. Relax.

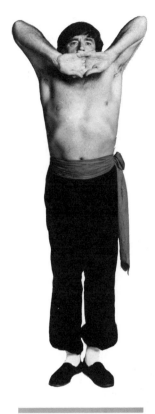

S T E P 5 ▲

Exhale steadily while reversing the movement exactly.

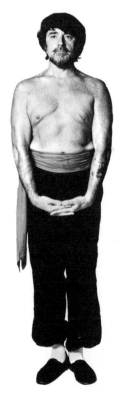

◄ **S T E P 6**

Back to the beginning position. Press down for the silent count of three. Repeat eight times.

The sixth exercise combines maximum upward stretching with maximum forward and downward stretching, hence the name. Take care if you have a back complaint.

THE BENEFIT Maximum stretching and bending combines arm and shoulder loosening, chest expansion, abdominal, back and leg exercise whilst greatly benefiting the kidneys and spleen.

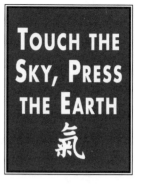

TOUCH THE SKY, PRESS THE EARTH
氣

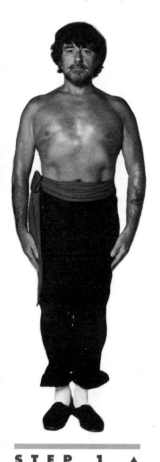

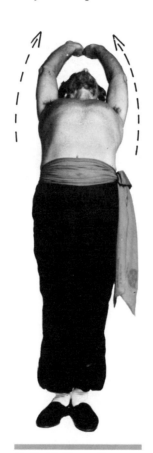

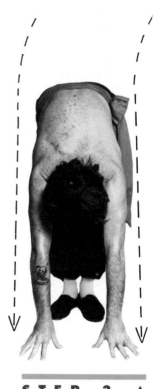

S T E P 1 ▲

Relax. Stand erect with feet together, hands loose at sides. Empty the lungs of air.

S T E P 2 ▲

Inhale slowly and deeply while raising the hands above the head and continuing a backward bend as far as possible. Hold for the silent count of three.

S T E P 3 ▲

Exhale steadily while reversing the movement forwards and downwards until the fingertips are pressed on the ground as far ahead of your toes as possible. Pause for the silent count of five.

STEP 4 ▼

Inhale slowly and deeply while straightening, drawing the hands up the legs to the thighs.

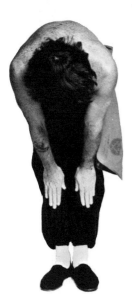

◀ STEP 5

Hold for the silent count of three.

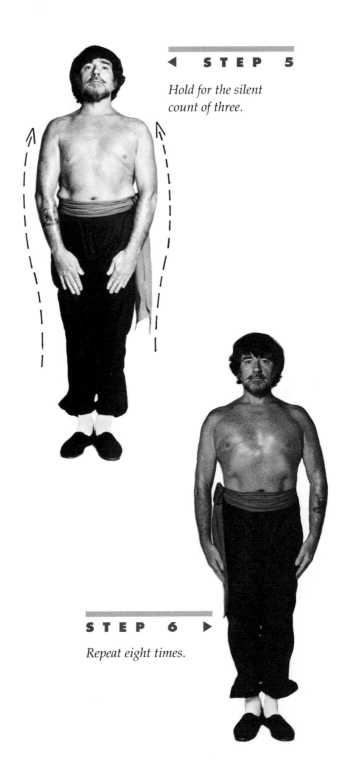

STEP 6 ▶

Repeat eight times.

The Seventh Exercise is perhaps so named because of the tiger's ability to look directly behind it while keeping its body poised for a frontal spring. We have all seen a cat stalking some unsuspecting prey, only to be disturbed by a sound or movement behind it. It will stop dead in its tracks, front paw raised, every muscle and sinew frozen in the direction of its chosen path, while turning its head to look directly back over its tail. Apparently, tigers do this also. Whatever the origin of its name, this seems as good an explanation as any, for it is just this action that the exercise calls for.

THE BENEFIT It loosens neck sinews, develops neck muscles, exercises the vital organs of the throat and promotes excellent balance while working calves, ankles and feet.

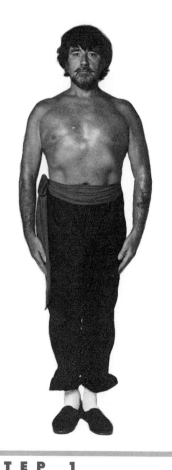

STEP 1 ▲

Relax. Stand erect with feet together, hands loose at sides. Empty the lungs of air.

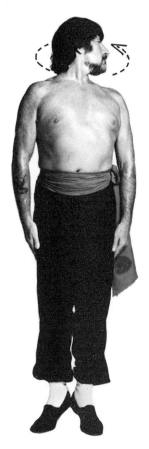

◀ **STEP 2**

Inhale slowly and deeply while gradually rising on the toes and turning the head as far to the left as possible. Do not turn the shoulders or upper body.

When the breath is complete, you should be fully raised on the toes, head twisted as far to the left as possible in an attempt to look behind you. Hold for the silent count of three.

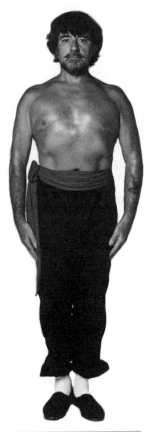

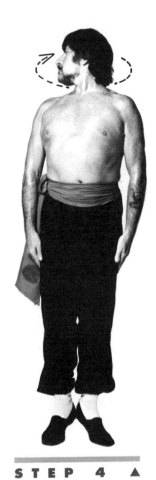

S T E P 3 ▲

*Exhale steadily while
reversing the movement
back to the starting
position.*

S T E P 4 ▲

*Repeat movement to the
right. Complete four
times on either side.*

The name of this eighth exercise is derived from the unique way of closing the fists. Each fist is fully formed yet leaves a hollow in its centre as though protecting a delicate object from being crushed. The fist, tensed to its full power when outstretched, must control the energy that surrounds the inner palm. This exercise develops a formidable hand grip, and greatly strengthens the arm while demanding passive control. It is one of the classic restraining movements, which, when released with full speed and impact after long practice, can unleash unbelievable but easily controlled force.

THE BENEFIT To increase power in the arms, from shoulder to elbow, to wrist, to fingers, is the main purpose; at the same time exercising the legs and lower trunk. It is in fact the 'slow motion' performance of the 'Kung Fu' punch with strict control on pressure and the restraint of energy. It is a little difficult to master and should be practised patiently and diligently from one stance at a time until ready to progress to the next. Pa Tuan Tsin only teaches the frontal punch, but I have included punching from the Right and Left Bow.

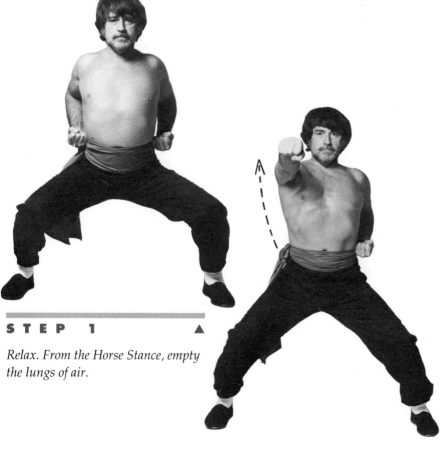

◄ STEP 2

Inhale slowly and deeply while extending the right fist in a frontal punch. The movement should begin from a relaxed shoulder, gradually increasing pressure as it turns and extends. When the fist is fully extended (imaginary swallow's egg safely shielded inside), tensed as if in a strike, the arm is also locked at the elbow, exerting full pressure. Hold for the silent count of three.

STEP 1 ▲

Relax. From the Horse Stance, empty the lungs of air.

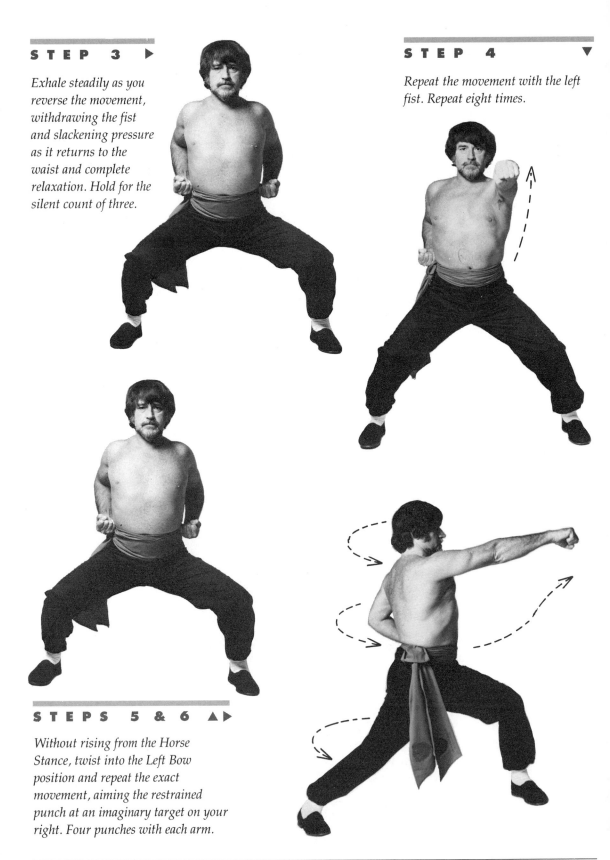

Exhale steadily as you reverse the movement, withdrawing the fist and slackening pressure as it returns to the waist and complete relaxation. Hold for the silent count of three.

Repeat the movement with the left fist. Repeat eight times.

Without rising from the Horse Stance, twist into the Left Bow position and repeat the exact movement, aiming the restrained punch at an imaginary target on your right. Four punches with each arm.

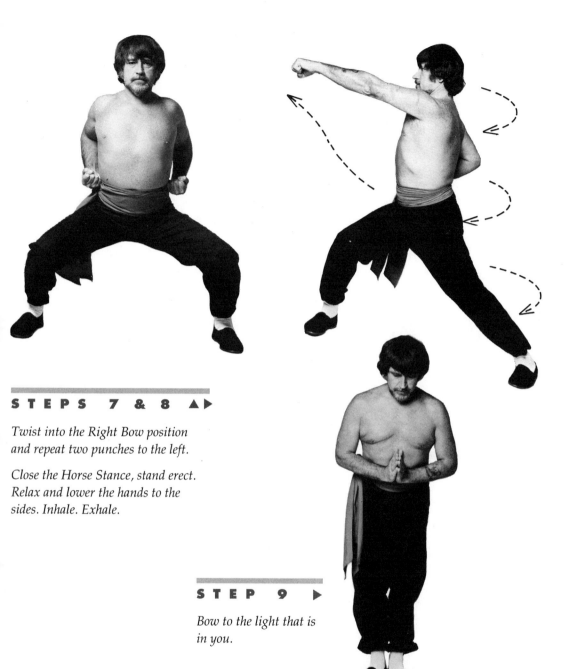

STEPS 7 & 8 ▲▶

Twist into the Right Bow position and repeat two punches to the left.

Close the Horse Stance, stand erect. Relax and lower the hands to the sides. Inhale. Exhale.

STEP 9 ▶

Bow to the light that is in you.

The final exercise of the Precious Eight may leave you a little wobbly at the knees, but otherwise feeling fine once you have closed the Horse Stance and straightened up. The temptation to sit down will also be great. Resist it. Ease tired leg muscles by walking about or, if you are practising in a room, just walk on the spot. Keep your legs moving for at least a five-minute period.

Sip some water or tea, allow your breathing to settle and become completely normal.

MAXIMUM BENEFITS

Now that the Eight Precious Sets of Exercises have been demonstrated there should be a few words about getting the maximum benefit out of your practice in the shortest time.

As with any routine, there will be those who make faster progress than others; some that are fitter or younger to begin with and take to it more naturally, and those who will find it more difficult to adapt to. The biggest danger, especially when learning from the words and pictures of a book without coaching or encouragement, is 'faith-lag', that drop in confidence in oneself and in the exercises that is bound to occur during the early stages of a forced discipline overseen by no one but yourself. How do we avoid the temptation to drop out? To start with, you would not have read this far unless you felt an interest or a need for some kind of improvement in your health. But that doesn't mean you will consider the contents without a certain amount of reservation.

As I have stressed at every opportunity, patience, discipline and willpower are the vital ingredients. Unlike many advertised 'get-fit' systems, these breathing exercises do not carry a money-back guarantee of a magnificent body in only seven days for just five minutes a day. They do not promise effortless, easy results that will neither interfere with your life nor take up your time. But, I repeat, they do offer at the very least definite, self-evident improvement in general fitness, increased strength and a degree of immunity from illness which might otherwise affect a less healthy body.

The various benefits to be had from Pa Tuan Tsin and the time taken to achieve them is entirely up to you, as is the ultimate goal of Ch'i. There is, however, a yardstick by which you can judge your progress and this also works as a guard against 'faith-lag'. Assuming you are able to adopt a daily routine (or at second best, every other day), the first four weeks will undoubtedly prove to be the dropping out period. You are very likely to find many of the exercises awkward and uncomfortable to execute in the beginning. Or, on the other hand, they may seem so easy that you will consider them meaningless. There will almost certainly be days when the last thing you will wish to contemplate is yourself in a pair of droopy pyjamas, poised unsteadily before a mirror, confronted by a neighbour's fence or a panorama of city rooftops; not to mention miserable weather and the possible indignities of a giggle or two from sceptical members of the household.

You will almost certainly find breath and body coordination difficult during the first few sessions. The combination of your mind, breathing and body movements may seem totally out of reach. That first month is the testing ground; the proving period that you must come through no matter how slowly, before you realise that you have begun.

It is best, then, to be aware of the normal stumbling blocks you can expect to encounter and how to deal with them. Firstly, do not hurry in your efforts to immediately follow the routine as laid out. It has been made clear that the warm-up exercises and extra exercises are not an essential part of the program, you may wish to leave them until you feel you want to include them.

You may even find it disheartening to try to follow the exact sequence of the exercises. Don't then. Study the stance and posture of each exercise separately, familiarise yourself with the feel of different movements and positions before attempting to coordinate them with your breathing. If a particular muscle or joint seems stubborn at a certain angle, be patient with it, massage it, coax it into position, test it tolerantly and be satisfied with the response until you feel it is ready for extra demands. You will very soon discover your body's capabilities and develop your own style.

Likewise with your breathing. As suggested earlier, practise it separately, concentrating first on prolonging and controlling the length and depth of your inhalation and exhalation by deep breathing as often as you can. Practise bypassing the lungs and reaching the diaphragm before applying breathing to body movement. Remember breathing can be practised at any time; in the car, walking the dog, at the office window, in bed or in the bath. You are always breathing, so why not practise breathing properly? Slowly and deeply through the nose.

You cannot always choose or influence the quality of the air you breathe and, of course, there are times and places when the shorter and shallower your respiration the better; in the wake of a diesel engine, for instance, in a particularly smoky bar or any closed-in and crowded area. Most of the time, however, there is nothing like slow, deep breathing to calm the nerves and liven up the step.

You will know when your breathing is improved, not only by its duration and depth but by its passage. You will find it cooling the back of your throat like a subdued rush of cold breeze rather than a scarcely noticed rhythm in the nostrils; your diaphragm will rise and fall rather than your chest and ribcage. This fresh awareness of breath is the first foothold in the climb to Ch'i and assures you that you are ready to apply it to Pa Tuan Tsin.

One last but very important word. Should you have any doubts whatever as to your physical capability to perform any of the exercises or should you find any one particularly difficult, it would be wise to take this book along to your doctor and ask for an opinion. This is particularly advisable if you are in poor health or suffering from any specific complaint.

If you decide that some of the exercises are not possible for you or just don't seem right, then drop them out of the sequence until you feel ready for them, adding them as you make progress or leaving them out all together.

The wonderful thing about Pa Tuan Tsin is that even if you were to practise only one of the exercises continually you would soon feel the benefit. Older Chinese, for instance, often have a favourite exercise and they practise it and nothing else every morning. The Shaolin Archer is one such gem. All over Hong Kong or any Chinese area in Asia you will see amahs and coolies, businessmen and shopkeepers, all drawing their imaginary bows in the first soft light of morning. Their Horse Stance may vary greatly in height and style, but they are all enjoying the same air.

An effective summary of the Chinese attitudes towards progress is contained in the following extract from my first Chin Wu examination report:

The perfection of your art lies in the difficult region between the heart's intent and the expression of this intent in gesture.
You know as well as we do where your problem is: in hesitation, in the lack of confidence in your stances and movements.
Perhaps your will to learn has surged ahead of your body's capacity to understand the lessons of the stances. You should learn to relax, to be kind and patient to your own body. Practise your forms in peace.
You have done better than you think.

EXTRA
EXERCISES

PART
SEVEN

These breathing exercises are for you to consider, to try out in your own way and in your own time, to find out which of them suits you best. It is unlikely that you will want to include them all in your daily routine – there wouldn't be the time and neither is there the need.

After trying all the exercises, many people just adopt the two or three sets of exercises they feel good about and make them an everyday habit. It is suggested you do the same. This does not mean you cannot learn and practise them all if you can. A very good idea is to spend a week practising one exercise only, then adding one more for another week to gradually increase until you have tried every exercise.

When you have discovered those you feel most comfortable with, you can alternate, giving yourself a variety of breathing workouts instead of concentrating on one set, which some people sooner or later may find boring. However you go about it, you should try to end up with the eight different sets of exercises you feel are right for you, follow the instructions as carefully as you can and try not to make modifications to suit yourself. These can be added to Pa Tuan Tsin or alternated to give a variety of exercises.

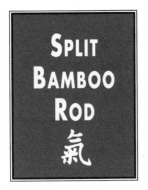

SPLIT BAMBOO ROD
氣

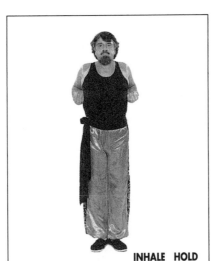

INHALE HOLD

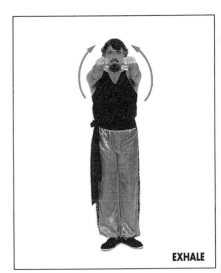

EXHALE

STEP 1 ▲

INHALATION *Stand straight with your feet together, hands loosely at your sides. Raise the fists to lower chest level — elbows in and pulled back with knuckles facing downward. Inhale slowly and deeply. Hold for the silent count of four to six seconds.*

STEP 2 ▲

EXHALATION *Slowly push your fists forward to arm's length, turning the knuckles upwards as your arms extend. Exhale slowly and silently in time with the movement.*

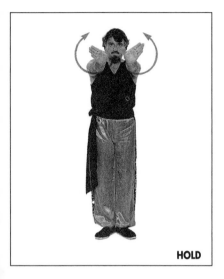

HOLD

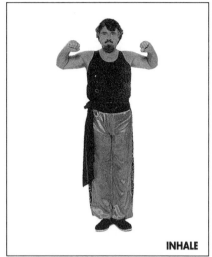

INHALE

STEP 3 ▲

With the breath expelled from the body, open the fists and perform a circular movement outwards with the fingers (as though splitting the imaginary bamboo rod) before closing the fists again.

STEP 4 ▲

INHALATION *Extend your arms slowly sideways until fully stretched (as though parting both halves of the imaginary bamboo rod). Bring the fists to shoulder level. Inhale slowly and deeply in time with the movement.*

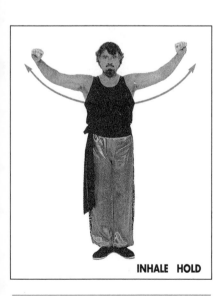

INHALE HOLD

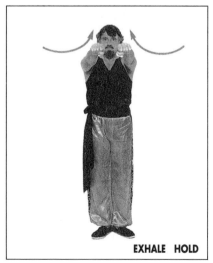

EXHALE HOLD

◄ STEP 6

EXHALATION *Slowly push your fists forwards (turning them as they extend) to arm's length (knuckles upward). Exhale slowly and silently in time with the movement. Repeat up to eight times.*

STEP 5 ▲

Complete movement of step 4.

OPEN TEMPLE GATES

气

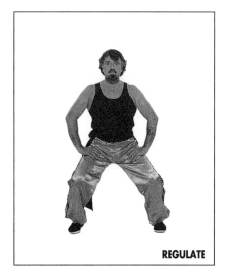

REGULATE

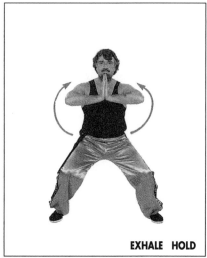

EXHALE HOLD

STEP 1 ▲

INHALATION *Open the horse stance,
half horse or full horse.*

STEP 2 ▲

*Press open palms together in the
prayer posture.*

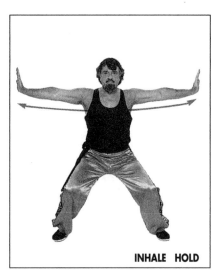

INHALE HOLD

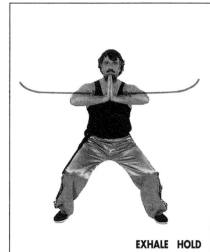

EXHALE HOLD

STEP 3 ▲

*Slowly extend your open palms to
each side to the full arm's extent, as
though pushing open the imaginary
gates. Inhale slowly and deeply in
time with the movement. Hold for the
silent count of four to six seconds.*

STEP 4 ▲

EXHALATION *Reverse the movement
until the open palms are again
pressed in the prayer posture.
Exhale slowly and silently in time
with movement. Repeat up to
eight times.*

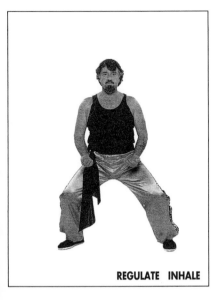

REGULATE INHALE

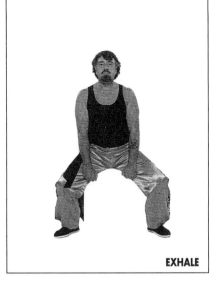

EXHALE

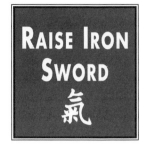

S T E P S   1 & 2   ▲

INHALATION *Regulate breathing with three to six normal breaths. Open the Horse Stance. Extend both arms downwards with your fists loosely closed, each grasping the hilt of an imaginary sword.*

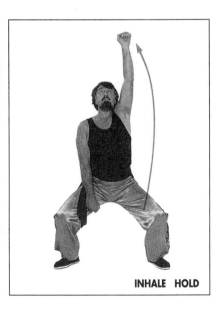

INHALE HOLD

◀   S T E P   3

Raise your left arm slowly outwards and upwards, keeping your elbow locked. Turn your head upwards in time with the movement, your eyes following the rising sword. Inhale deeply on the upward movement. Hold for the silent count of four to six seconds.

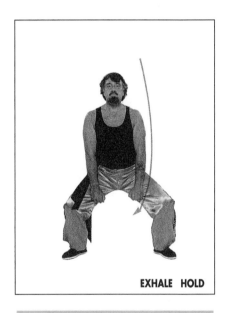

EXHALE HOLD

S T E P   4   ▲

EXHALATION *Slowly lower your left arm, your head lowering with the movement. Exhale silently in time with the movement. Hold for the silent count of four to six seconds.*

STEP 5 ▶

INHALATION *Raise your right arm slowly outwards and upwards, keeping the elbow locked. Turn your head upwards in time with the movement, your eyes following the rising sword. Inhale deeply on the upwards movement. Hold for the silent count of four to six seconds.*

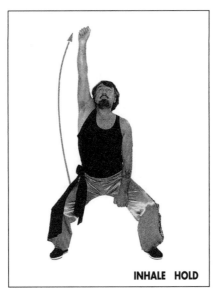

INHALE HOLD

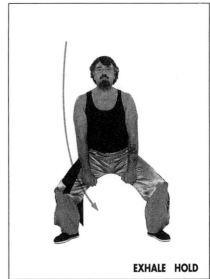

EXHALE HOLD

STEP 6 ▲

EXHALATION *Slowly lower your right arm, your head lowering with the movement. Exhale silently in time with the movement. Hold for the silent count of four to six seconds. Repeat up to four times each side.*

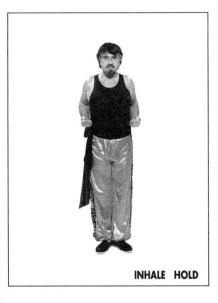

INHALE HOLD

◀ **S T E P 1**

INHALATION *Stand erect with your feet together, your fists level with your lower chest, the elbows in and back. Inhale slowly and deeply. Hold for the silent count of four to six seconds.j*

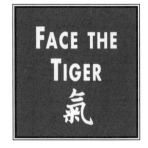

FACE THE TIGER
氣

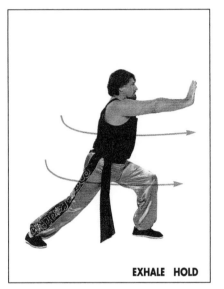

EXHALE HOLD

◀ **S T E P 2**

EXHALATION *Turn your head to face left and form the Left Bow Stance. Extend both hands to the left, palms outwards repelling the imaginary tiger. Exhale silent in time with the movement. Hold for the silent count of four to six seconds.*

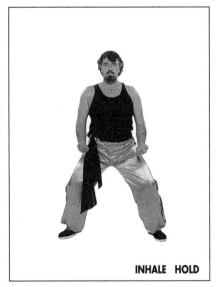

INHALE HOLD

S T E P 3 ▲

INHALATION *Return to the Horse Stance. Inhale slowly and deeply. Hold for the silent count of four to six seconds.*

EXHALE HOLD

◀ **S T E P 4**

EXHALATION *Reverse the movement — turn your head to the right and form the Right Bow Stance. Extend both hands to the right, palms outwards repelling the imaginary tiger. Exhale silently in time with the movement. Hold for the silent count of four to six seconds. Repeat up to four times each side.*

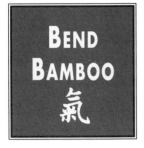

BEND BAMBOO
氣

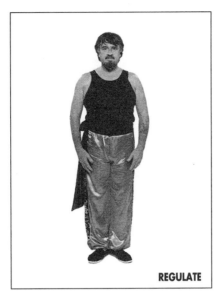

REGULATE

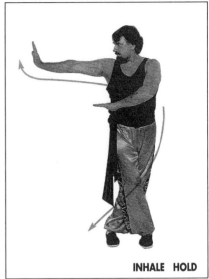

INHALE HOLD

STEP 1 ▲

INHALATION *Regulate breathing with three to six normal breaths. Stand straight with your feet together and your hands loosely at your sides.*

STEP 2 ▲

Cross your right leg over the left leg and stand firmly. Extend your right arm to full length, palm facing outwards, head facing right. Cross your left arm over your lower chest at the same time, palm downwards. Inhale deeply in time with the movement.

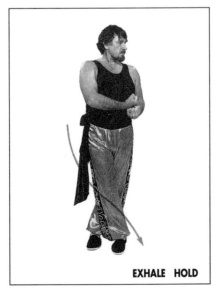

EXHALE HOLD

◄ STEP 3

EXHALATION *Close your right fist over the imaginary bamboo. Slowly draw in the right fist beside the stationary left fist. Exhale silently in time with the movement. Hold for the silent count of four to six seconds.*

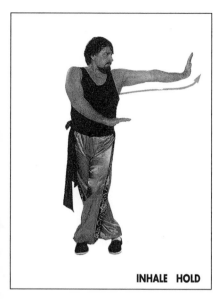

INHALE HOLD

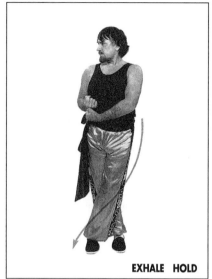

EXHALE HOLD

S T E P   4   ▲

INHALATION *Reverse the movement —
cross your left leg over your right leg
and stand firmly. Extend your left
arm to full length, palm facing away
and your head facing left. Cross your
right arm over your lower chest,
palm downwards. Inhale deeply
in time with the movement. Hold
for the silent count of four to
six seconds.*

S T E P   5   ▲

EXHALATION *Close your left fist over
the imaginary bamboo. Slowly draw
in the left fist beside the stationary
right fist. Exhale silently in time
with the movement. Hold for the
silent count of four to six seconds.
Repeat up to four times each side.*

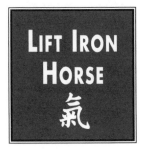

LIFT IRON HORSE
氣

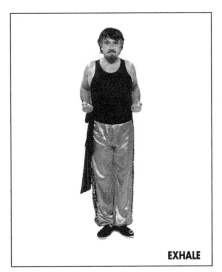

EXHALE

INHALATION*Stand straight with your fists at hip level.*

STEPS 2, 3 & 4

Lower your hands to your sides then raise them into the prayer posture, palms pressed together, fingertips at lip level. Push your hands outwards to arm's length, then upwards to meet, palms together, above your head in a sweeping movement. Inhale slowly and deeply in time with the movement. Inhale slowly and deeply in time with the movement. Hold for the silent count of four to six seconds.

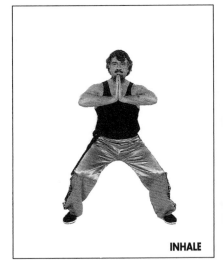

INHALE

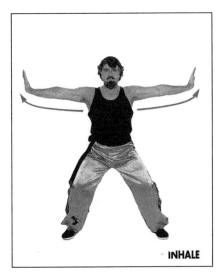

INHALE

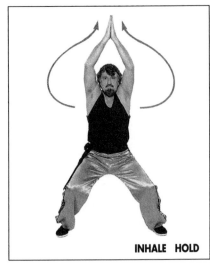

INHALE HOLD

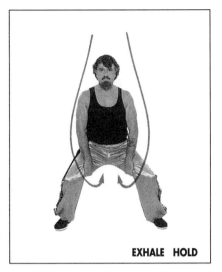

EXHALE HOLD

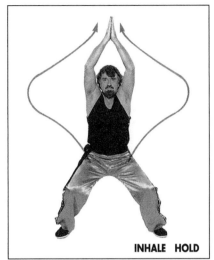

INHALE HOLD

STEP 5 ▲

EXHALATION *Allow your hands to descend until they grasp each thigh firmly (as though trying to lift yourself from the Horse Stance). Pull upwards with a definite pull on the thighs, as though forcing the last gram of breath from your body. Exhale silently in time with the movement.*

STEP 6 ▲

INHALATION *Remain in the Horse Stance and repeat the first movement — outwards and upwards to the prayer posture above the head. Inhale slowly and deeply in time with the movement. Hold for the silent count of four to six seconds.*

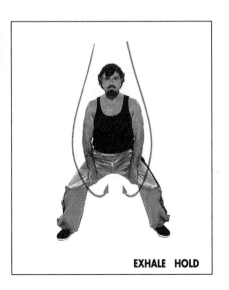

EXHALE HOLD

◄ STEP 7

EXHALATION *Repeat the second movement — allow hands to descend and grasp the thighs firmly, pull upwards as though trying to lift your weight from the Horse Stance. Exhale silently for the count of four to six seconds. Repeat up to eight times.*

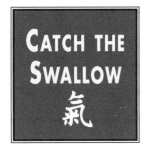

CATCH THE SWALLOW

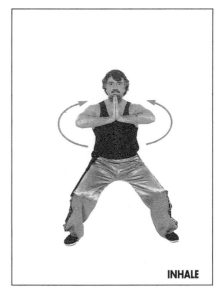

REGULATE

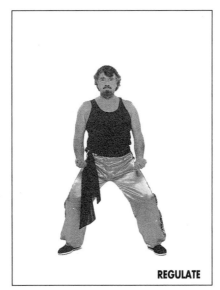

INHALE

STEPS 1, 2, 3 & 4

INHALATION *Open the Horse Stance. Press your palms together in the prayer posture. Extend your arms outwards with your palms facing outwards. Raise your arms above the head and bring your palms back together in the prayer posture, catching the tail of the imaginary swallow. Inhale slowly and deeply in time with the movement. Hold for the silent count of four to six seconds.*

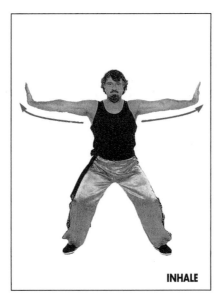

INHALE

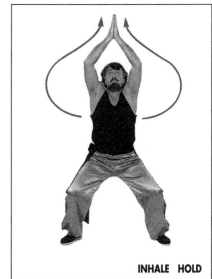

INHALE HOLD

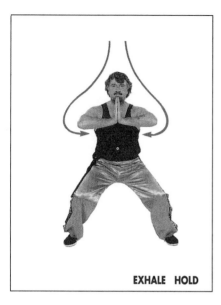

EXHALE HOLD

EXHALATION *Draw your pressed palms slowly downwards to their original position. Exhale slowly and silently in time with the movement. Hold for the silent count of four to six seconds. Repeat up to eight times.*

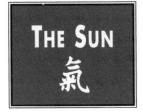

THE SUN
气

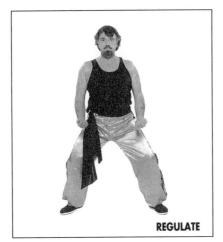

REGULATE

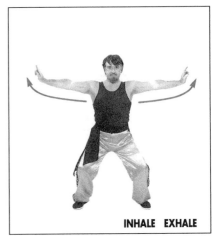

INHALE   EXHALE

STEPS 1 & 2 ▲

INHALATION *Form the Horse Stance. Slowly stretch your arms outwards, figures lightly closed, forefinger raised (the imaginary sun sets). Inhale deeply in time with the movement. Hold the position for the silent count of eight to ten seconds as you exhale.*

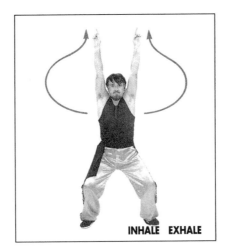

INHALE   EXHALE

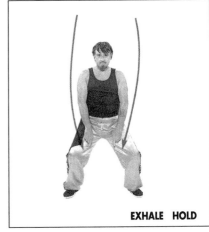

EXHALE   HOLD

STEP 3 ▲

INHALATION *Raise your outstretched arms sideways above your head, fingers pointing skywards (the sun rises). Inhale deeply in time with the movement. Hold for the silent count of eight to ten seconds.*

STEP 4 ▲

EXHALATION *Lower your outstretched arms forwards until the fingers are pointing earthwards (the suns sets). Exhale silently in time with movement. Hold for the silent count of eight to ten seconds. Repeat all three movements four times.*

ADVANCED
EXERCISES

Breath is the Emperor and the mind is the Prime Minister.
Breath is active in sleep whereas the mind is not.

Hindu saying

PART
EIGHT

The following exercises are not a part of Pa Tuan Tsin but they are recommended for those who can find the time and stamina to fit them in. Perhaps begin to include them as you become further advanced. Each of them is part of the Wu Shu exercise routine and designed to improve the circulation of Ch'i. They are not so much breathing exercises but rather exercises for strengthening the legs, arms and hands.

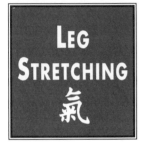

LEG STRETCHING
气

First, the simple process of stretching the legs and bending at the waist, in much the same way as a ballet dancer practises on a wall bar. If you don't have a bar, the garden fence or an improvisation will do.

Start with the bar at a comfortable (but not too comfortable) height — at least waist high. Raise the right leg until the heel is resting upon the bar with the leg absolutely straight. Left leg rigid, locked at the knee, toe at 12 o'clock.

This exercise really puts the muscles and tendons in the backs of the legs to work. Don't be surprised or concerned if you experience soreness, it will soon disappear. Leg stretching will also help you in the bending exercises of Pa Tuan Tsin.

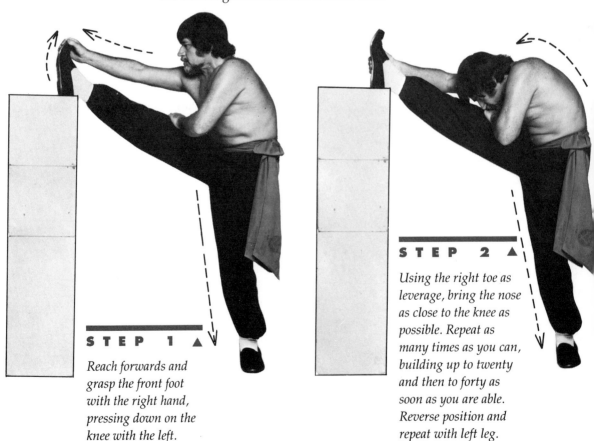

STEP 1 ▲

Reach forwards and grasp the front foot with the right hand, pressing down on the knee with the left.

STEP 2 ▲

Using the right toe as leverage, bring the nose as close to the knee as possible. Repeat as many times as you can, building up to twenty and then to forty as soon as you are able. Reverse position and repeat with left leg.

After a session of leg stretching, the overwhelming urge is to bend them. Simple squats executed slowly bring instant relief to stretched legs and complete the natural movement.

Reverse the movement by slowly rising and lowering the arms while inhaling slowly and deeply on the way up. Repeat as many times as comfortable (try for five and increase with progress).

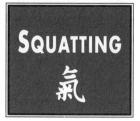

SQUATTING

氣

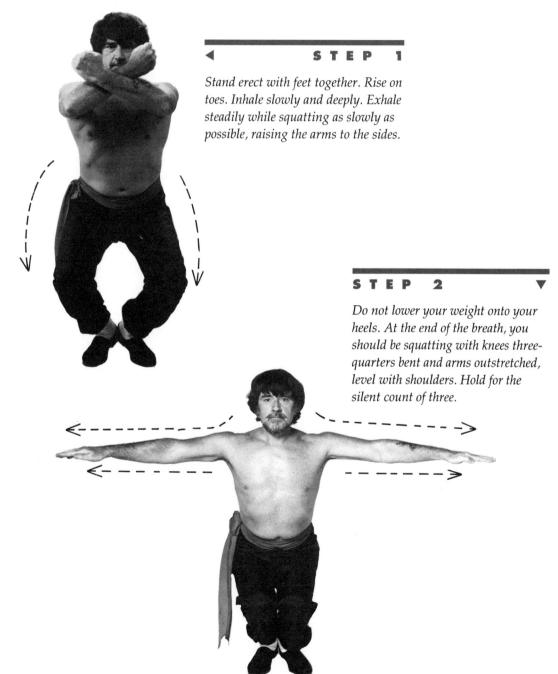

◄ **S T E P   1**

Stand erect with feet together. Rise on toes. Inhale slowly and deeply. Exhale steadily while squatting as slowly as possible, raising the arms to the sides.

S T E P   2 ▼

Do not lower your weight onto your heels. At the end of the breath, you should be squatting with knees three-quarters bent and arms outstretched, level with shoulders. Hold for the silent count of three.

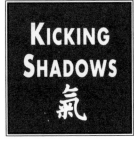

KICKING SHADOWS
氣

Apart from the striking power developed by such leg exercises, Kicking Shadows is a very effective way to try out these new legs of yours. And after six weeks of practising the Horse Stance, you will indeed have new legs.

There are many kicks for the Wu Shu practitioner to develop: side, back and front, performed from standing, squatting, lying, or from midair, often a good 2 metres above the ground. These highly dangerous and difficult lightning strikes with the feet are perhaps the most breathtaking and incredible manifestations of the power of Ch'i in the advanced Wu Shu student. They are far beyond the reach of the average healthy and athletic person and, of course, are best left alone by all but the serious martial artist.

I have chosen the two most simple but effective strike kicks, emphasising that they are suggested as an excellent addition to your Pa Tuan Tsin practice. They are offered only to speed up the reflexes and to test and increase leg power. They are also an excellent way of letting off steam when the spirit of Ch'i is at its height.

It must be emphasised that their use as a strike, even in defence, should be avoided at all costs unless you are under the supervision of a recognised Kung Fu instructor. Even then he/she will advise against their use unless in deadly combat. Frontal kicks, both high and low (throat/chest, groin/knee) can not only cause serious injury or death, they can also put the kicker at a total balance disadvantage unless an expert.

NOTE You may find either of these kicking techniques difficult to cultivate as demonstrated and if so dispense with the Bow position and the target of the hand. Simply practise the kicks from the stand punch position with knees half bent until you have developed the balance and the knack.

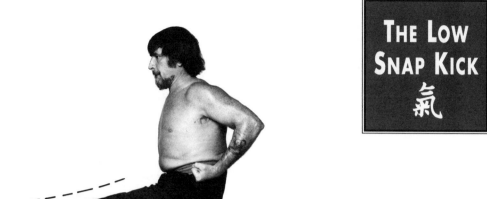

THE LOW SNAP KICK

气

STEP 1

Feet together, knees slightly bent, hands firmly in punch position. Inhale.

STEP 2 ▲

Raise the left knee and snap the foot out from the waist with a whip-like action, making sure the striking foot is stretched in line with the leg.

THE HIGH SNAP KICK

气

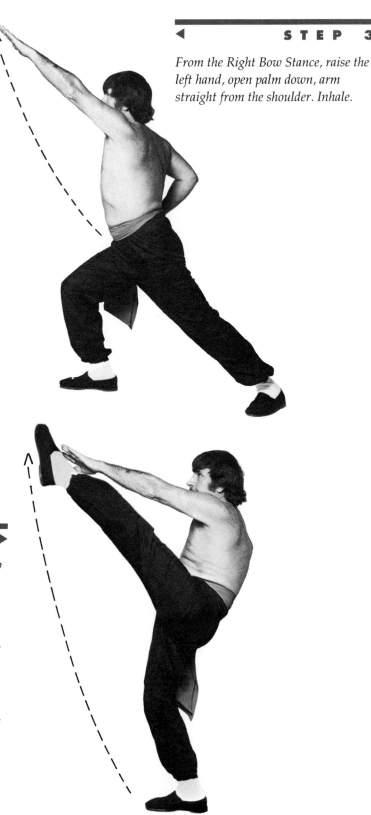

◄ **STEP 3**

From the Right Bow Stance, raise the left hand, open palm down, arm straight from the shoulder. Inhale.

STEP 4 ►

Bend the left leg at the knee and snap it out to strike the raised palm with the outstretched foot. As soon as the strike is made, return the leg to its Bow Position. Speed, power and stability are the purpose; accuracy of aim and contact will come with practice. As you progress, repeat the low kick as many times as you are able (aim for ten). Reverse to the Left Bow and repeat with the right foot. This is, of course, more difficult to perform, perhaps impossible, if you are not including leg stretching in your routine.

An exercise in agility and flexibility, this and similar classic postures are widely used in several forms of Wu Shu. Basically a feinting manoeuvre, it leaves an opponent with the impression of retreat while actually avoiding a leg attack or dodging a fist strike and positioning for an unexpectedly low counterattack.

For our purpose, however, it is merely a satisfying culmination for all your patient leg work. It may take you some time to achieve it comfortably and steadily, but achieve it you will. It is perhaps the ultimate leg exercise when all other work has prepared you for it.

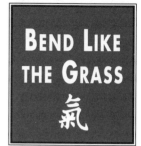

BEND LIKE THE GRASS
氣

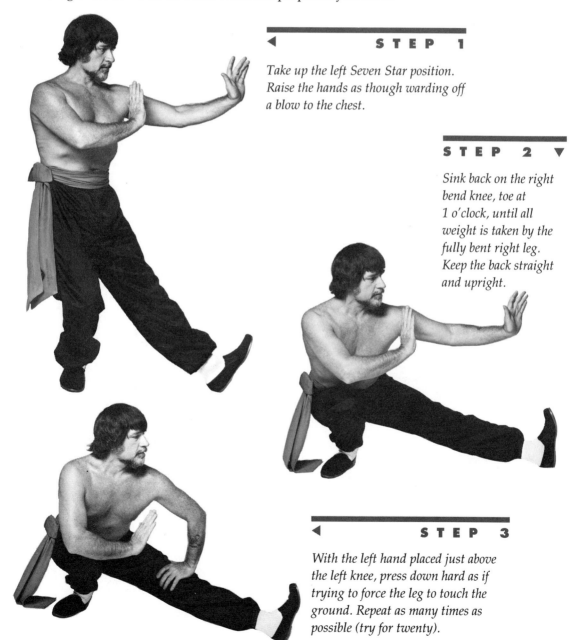

◄ STEP 1

Take up the left Seven Star position. Raise the hands as though warding off a blow to the chest.

STEP 2 ▼

Sink back on the right bend knee, toe at 1 o'clock, until all weight is taken by the fully bent right leg. Keep the back straight and upright.

◄ STEP 3

With the left hand placed just above the left knee, press down hard as if trying to force the leg to touch the ground. Repeat as many times as possible (try for twenty).

This is a difficult manoeuvre for anyone whose hips and lower joints are unaccustomed to regular exercise and it should only be attempted in the sixth week of practice. It is likely that at first you will lose balance, find yourself unable to 'get down' all the way and feel far from dignified. You will discover though, that you can get a little lower, a little more stable, upright and comfortable each day, until it is a pleasure to reach and hold with ease. A quiet conclusion to your months of patience, determination and discipline.

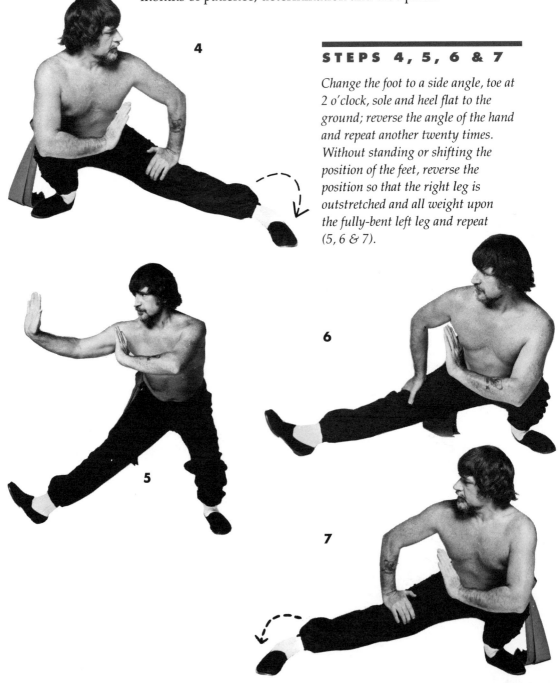

STEPS 4, 5, 6 & 7

Change the foot to a side angle, toe at 2 o'clock, sole and heel flat to the ground; reverse the angle of the hand and repeat another twenty times. Without standing or shifting the position of the feet, reverse the position so that the right leg is outstretched and all weight upon the fully-bent left leg and repeat (5, 6 & 7).

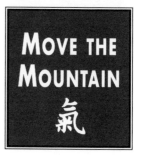

MOVE THE MOUNTAIN
氣

Move the Mountain is a classic Tiger Claw exercise. Although somewhat modified for our poses, it develops power in the arms and shoulders while giving the benefit of the Horse Stance, increasing lung capacity and improving circulation. The Chinese believe this exercise has excellent recuperative effects and use it to round off a heavy training session or to wind down after a bout of free sparring. It is an ideal way to complete your practice.

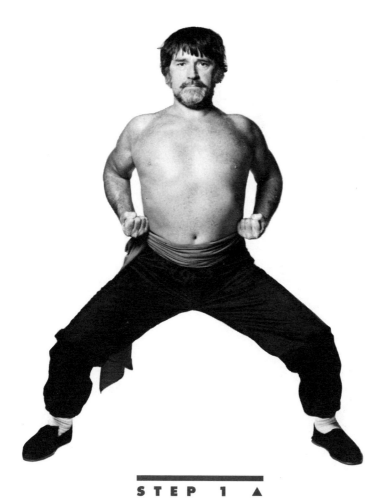

STEP 1 ▲

Open the Horse Stance.

◀ **S T E P 2**

*Inhale fully, bringing
the arms up and elbows
back until the hands are
beside the shoulders,
palms facing out and
forefingers pointing up.*

◀ **S T E P 3**

*Exhale slowly and steadily as the
hands are very gradually pushed
forward in line with the knees. Force
is concentrated along the arms to the
fingertips as though rolling a boulder
from the mouth of a cave that
imprisons you. At the end of the
breath every ounce of strength and
mental concentration should be
directed to the fingertips, arms
stretched to their fullest and held for
the count of three.*

*Exhale slowly and steadily while
relaxing the arms and withdrawing
them back to the shoulder position.
Hold for the count of three and repeat
eight times.*

Western Health Practices Compatible with Ch'i

Part Nine

Exercising
and Ch'i

The exercises in this book are directed to all those who could be affected by any of the common afflictions of modern living but care, and above all patience, is emphasised at every stage. For these reasons, it is suggested that improved breathing habits alone are not enough. While they can and will go far to improve wellbeing, improvement will be more definitely and quickly achieved with the help of compatible exercises aimed at stretching and strengthening muscles to improve flexibility, and relaxation techniques to prepare the nervous system and calm the mind for the concentration that is part of Chi Kung.

Energy balance — Yin and Yang — should be an important part of Chi Kung training, so nutrition can greatly affect your ability to make progress. These important additions to the program of exercises are suggested later in the book.

If you follow the rules of basic Chi Kung carefully, with proper attention to compatible exercise and nutrition, and providing you practise fairly regularly at least, you can expect to feel increasingly lighter, fitter, more relaxed and far more energetic than you did when you decided to begin.

If you were to join an authentic Chinese Kung Fu school, breathing exercises would probably be the first thing you would be taught. But they would be taught in conjunction with other carefully considered training methods designed to condition the body inside and out. You would be taught stances to strengthen the legs for endurance, agility and balance. Certain basic stances are considered a vital part of the development of Ch'i. Practice and perfection of the stance go hand-in-hand with practice and perfection of the generation and circulation of Ch'i power.

So important did the old Masters consider the basic stances that the stringency of their methods of teaching them is legendary. A new student was and still is judged by the ability to conquer the stances and endure them for long periods, so that when called upon in combat the power is there and the reserve endless.

Some stories claim serious students were taught to Horse Stance and sent away to practise it for up to three years before being judged ready to continue.

The stance than, is practised to keep one upright, steady and nimble on the feet, but all other parts of the body are also carefully and systematically considered. With the internal organs, bones and sinews nourished by Chi Kung, the muscles and joints are put through the 'Chen Tao' repeated routines of stress and stretch, block and strike, squat and leap, advance and retreat, while the mind is exercised by memorising scores of intricate and exacting movements of up to seventy and eighty variations and imagining their application to an opponent. Constantly drilled and re-drilled until body and mind work as one, reflexes are immediate and responses accurate.

As this book is not for the martial arts enthusiast, we cannot expect or aspire to the rigours and benefits of martial arts training. If we are to practise its basic stances and some of its breathing exercises, however, we must also develop our own compatible routine to support them. Improved health will not come without the three essentials — *exercise*, *nutrition* and *relaxation*. One without the other is a waste of time and a frustration that can be worse than no effort at all.

With Chi Kung as its main purpose, our programme must also condition the body through other exercise — physical exertion that will depend on the right fuel to give it energy through eating and drinking. Not necessarily the confusing and highly debatable effects of fad dieting or the extremes of vegetarianism, but at least an awareness of what to eat and drink: when to eat it and drink it; what foods and liquids are good for us and why, what are bad for us and why; what foods and liquids complement each other and which ones destroy or neutralise each other. In other words, basic commonsense nutrition.

There are no secrets or revelations, no sudden discoveries of wonder foods that by simply being swallowed will give us renewed strength and vigour. In fact what discoveries there are came from the distant past: the discovery of natural foods organically grown and untouched by chemical agents. But of course it's not quite that easy. We may take the trouble to find out what natural foods are best for us and vow never again to touch anything else, but finding a regular supply is another question.

As demand grows so does the need for volume and with volume comes mass processing, artificial flavourings, preservatives and forced agriculture which depletes soil and therefore grains, fruits and vegetables — and even meat, poultry and eggs — of vital organic properties, creating the need for supplements of vitamins and minerals in pill and capsule form.

The third essential is relaxation, the ability to conquer or at least learn to live with stress, the pressures put upon us by the events that pattern our everyday lives. Again there are no new discoveries, except in the synthetic and negative form of prescription drugs developed to give temporary relief. Again, what discoveries are made take the form of the rediscovery of age-old practices of meditation and methods of relaxation originating in the Oriental past.

So, when we consider the practice of Chi Kung we must also consider the practice, to some degree, of these three other essentials: compatible 'Western' exercise, basic nutrition and methods of relaxation — one is wasted without the support of the others.

You cannot successfully develop a powerful Ch'i without a reasonably healthy body. You cannot expect a healthy body without considering what you eat and drink. You cannot benefit from either without the ability to relax. Suggestions for these three essential elements will be made through the later pages of this book.

Before laying out our Chi Kung programme let us look first at the question of other exercise. Outside the Kung Fu school the Chinese approach to exercise is a studied and rather low-key one, particularly among older people. Comparative poverty and hard physical work have always been an accepted part of ordinary Chinese life, so the quest for intense and regular exercise is neither as popular nor as necessary as it is in the West. Not that there is any less interest in self-preservation, in fact the average Chinese of any position in life is probably more consistent in affairs of basic health than his or her Western counterpart.

To the Chinese, the secret of a long and healthy life is consistency. No matter how modest the exercise routine may be, it must be performed every day regardless of age, weather or even poor health. It is a matter of habit and unless bedridden or forbidden by a doctor they will exercise, perhaps not always well, wisely or effectively, but consistently.

This does not suggest every Chinese is a picture of health and fitness or free from sickness, but whatever else gets in their way the regular practice of their individual ritual is never forgotten. If a Master even suspects his student of skipping the daily training practice the offender is marked as a potential failure and asked to leave the school if the irregularity continues.

Of course, Chinese youth as a whole is very sports and exercise minded, tending to replace the traditional 'soft' style of physical conditioning with the harder, more modern and less flowing track and field athletics, racquet games, gymnastics, and weight training as well as the traditional martial arts. Those who cannot afford the luxury of such endeavours are likely to be engaged in such hard labour that added exercise is the last thing they need.

We in the West are in a different situation. Hard, sustained physical labour is rare and becoming rarer. Even physical work itself is affected by advanced technology. We are more likely to be seated behind a desk, a computer or a word processor with little time and less opportunity to walk our songbirds or take the air beneath our favourite tree as a start to each and every day.

WHAT'S RIGHT FOR YOU

The practice of breathing exercise alone, although it will improve your health, is not enough. It will not give you the kind of pulse-rising activity your body needs to perform properly unless you do something more. But before choosing from the many forms of exercise that are open to you, from the group involvement of aerobic dancing, jazzercise, competitive sport or jogging or walking alone, consider carefully. The wrong exercise at the wrong time for the wrong purpose can do more harm than good.

Once you have accepted the fact that some form of physical activity is essential for toning and firming muscles, improving the cardiovascular system, increasing the flow of blood and oxygen through the body to bring nutrients to vital organs and help eliminate waste, the next step is to determine which exercise is best for you. No two of us are quite the same, so the choice of the conditioning routine to go with your breathing exercises should be considered very carefully.

Westerners of all ages, both sexes and from all locations and walks of life are out there pounding the pavements and parks of cities and suburbs to lose weight, to build up, to trim down; to strengthen the heart, get rid of tension or simply to show how good they look in Reeboks and running shorts.

Gym junkies have created a whole new race of fanatics who make the fitness centre their second home and sports store owners rich and happy. They work out whether they are up to it or not, often pursuing the wrong exercise in the wrong way.

Determined converts who are not really 'morning people' are climbing sleepily onto exercise bikes and forcing themselves through excruciating minutes with one eye on the clock and the other on the coffee pot. The health revolution has anyone who is reasonably active and suitably determined — and some that aren't — pumping iron and pitting themselves against weights and pulleys in the fitness club, pulling on running shoes or returning squash balls as though they were deadly missiles.

For far too many, the result is a range of sports injuries stemming from overexercise, wrong exercise or the right exercise wrongly applied.

AVOID RISK OF INJURY

Sports medicine is a comparatively new science that has developed along with the advancement of competitive and recreational sport and the increasing concern with physical fitness. Injury manifests itself more and more as more and more people of all types and ages — in all manner of physical condition — seek to improve themselves with weight training and other unaccustomed activities in often overcrowded fitness centres and spasmodic bursts of jogging or aerobic activity.

Even those gyms and well-run centres with knowledgeable and professionally attentive instructors are hard pressed to keep an eye on beginners once the brief and sometimes sketchy initiation sessions are over and the exerciser is left to his or her own devices. Poor instruction, misinterpretation or simple overenthusiasm can lead to debilitating strains, sprains and muscle tears that can discourage and frustrate the most determined beginner.

Published medical research can be confusing when it comes to getting and staying fitter; no sooner has one enlightening fact been discovered than it is eclipsed by another. What's good for us today is suddenly suspect tomorrow.

For instance, leading American cardiologists suggest that vigorous exercise cannot in itself prevent or cure heart disease. Fitness, they say, is defined by the capacity for hard physical activity and endurance. It is a measure of functional ability. It doesn't necessarily reflect the presence or absence of disease and implies nothing about the actual condition of the arteries or the heart. They also warn that stress tests will not necessarily detect symptoms of coronary heart disease and a normal cardiograph is not always evidence of a clean bill of cardiovascular health.

Other research has shown that the pleasures of easygoing social interaction and the soothing, down-to-earth enjoyment of pets are forms of natural medicine. Walks in the open air, the pursuit of hobbies such as gardening, fishing, bushwalking or just sitting down to a good read, all the simpler aspects of life, can often do more for the human heart than the most brilliant surgeon.

On the other hand, these fairly obvious findings don't indicate that a walk around the block with Fido, a passing chat with Mrs Brown next door or a few chapters of James Herriot will guarantee a longer, healthier life. We must also work to rid ourselves of the unhappiness and frustration of stress if we want to achieve and maintain good health.

Our bodies were not made for indolence, they were designed for action. If we get caught up in the comfort and convenience of modern living — driving when we could walk, sitting when we could stand, avoiding the unpleasantness of breathlessness or perspiration, we'll soon find even a flight of stairs a formidable obstacle. Later on in life, walking or even standing will begin to seem an effort best done without.

Although you may be able to say, 'But I've never smoked or drunk alcohol and I've always been careful of what I eat', that is only a start: it is not enough without some form of exercise. The need will differ from case to case, and men's and women's situations too can be quite different. As a rule, the activity of a wife and mother requires a lot of energy and a great deal of physical labour. Even a professional woman will have a home as well as a job and a social life to maintain — plus a powerhouse of female hormones that seem to keep cardiovascular deterioration at bay, even in sedentary office workers, at least until middle age.

It is inactivity in women over fifty that often causes them to suffer from predictable ailments of middle age such as high blood pressure and diabetes as much as their male counterparts. Once inactivity has set in, we can soon become too weak to lift anything, walk to the shops or approach a flight of steps with anything but weariness. Our posture suffers, we don't like what we see in the mirror, our self-esteem is affected and before we know where we are, we are feeling and looking older than we should. So what can we do about it?

Perhaps the most acceptable suggestion to those of us who have never enjoyed exercise and feel we never will, is that a little regular attention to our body and its function is better than none at all.

Breathing exercises are probably the best choice of all for the unenthusiastic. The comparatively gentle practice of Chi Kung breathing will help earn us life's little luxuries and maintain a stable level of well-being in spite of indulgences such as a few drinks or even cigarettes.

Choosing compatible exercise is up to you, but here are some thoughts and suggestions to help condition both body and mind towards maintaining it.

GOOD REASONS FOR EXERCISE

Without exercise, the body quite simply deteriorates through lack of use.

- Muscles get thinner and weaker until they slacken entirely.
- The heart gets smaller and therefore more vulnerable with time.
- The joints stiffen up and invite complaints such as arthritis.
- The lungs are less able to take in air and our breathing gets shorter and more difficult.

If you are fit, you wake up better prepared to face whatever the day will bring. Your capacity for work will be improved. You will not tire so easily. You will be less prone to irritability.

HOW YOUR BODY REACTS

When you exercise properly, the muscles, including the heart, get bigger and stronger. The bigger heart can pump more blood and so it beats more slowly and is therefore less stressed. An efficient heart means an efficient body. The capacity of the lungs increases to take in more air with each breath, putting more oxygen into the bloodstream. The joints stay mobile so you can twist and turn and bend without effort through a full range of movement.

EXERCISE AND CHOLESTEROL

Exercise increases the circulation of the blood, millions of new red blood corpuscles emerge from the bone marrow and join the bloodstream to revive tired blood. Concentrations of fatty substances in your blood (cholesterol and triglycerides) are reduced, which lessens the danger of arterial blockage from blood clots.

These effects will make the practice of breathing exercises easier for you and help the steady development of your Ch'i.

HOW TO BEGIN?

First of all, you don't have to aspire to athletic achievement in order to develop and maintain reasonable physical condition. Fifteen to twenty minutes a day is all it takes, provided those valuable minutes are used wisely and properly.

If every day is more than your schedule or motivation will allow, then at least three times a week reasonably spaced — say Mondays, Wednesdays and Fridays or Tuesdays, Thursdays and Saturdays either included in your Chi Kung programme or separate from it. As long as the pattern is regular it will begin to form a cycle that the body will become used to. The ruin of any exercise routine is inconsistency.

HOW HARD SHOULD YOU TRY?

If you are the type who becomes easily bored with exercise you can overcome that tendency to a degree by alternating between breathing exercises and other related conditioning activity, whether it is gym work, racquet games, golf, swimming, skipping (if you're fit enough) or simply energetic walking.

Any of these will elevate your pulse rate and get the blood flowing along with your newfound Ch'i. All you need to tell you it is working is a light sweat and to be slightly out of breath. If you cannot find breath to talk or whistle during such activity, you are overdoing it.

If you prefer the comparatively passive stretching methods of Hatha Yoga or light callisthenics, either will be very compatible with Chi Kung.

Surely it isn't too much to ask for, say, twenty minutes of your day to maintain and protect the most valuable possession you have. On the other hand, if your enthusiasm puts you into the fanatical class, don't overdo things. If you choose weight training, allow forty-eight hours between workouts. Take off at least one day a week without exercise of any significant kind to allow minor muscle tissue tears to rebuild and restore their supply of energy-giving glycogen.

However you decide to approach it, make sure the method is suited to your type, age, and state of fitness and health to begin with. The following chart can help you decide. If it seems painfully obvious, you are no doubt among those people who are already accustomed to exercise. Remind yourself of the Chinese way — consider every aspect of the action you contemplate and take into account its advantages and disadvantages to the entire system.

HOW LONG SHOULD YOU EXERCISE?

1 If you have not exercised regularly for, say, at least a month, take things easy, treat yourself gently. If you go in headfirst, you could pull a muscle or strain a ligament that will stop you before you start.
2 Check with your doctor, particularly if you are over forty, for the following:
♦ How is your blood pressure? Low or high?
♦ If you are a heavy smoker, how has it affected your respiratory system?
♦ Are you overweight, say, more than 7 to 10 kilograms?
♦ If you're not accustomed to exercise, how does your doctor rate your capacity?
♦ Have you any history of heart disease or any other serious illness. Should it be taken into consideration?
♦ Are you subject to any stress-related illness or condition such as hypertension, migraine, headache, muscular tension, joint or back pains, dizziness or sleeping problems? If so, should you modify your exercise plan accordingly?
   Do not feel your body has let you down if you are told to adjust slowly and carefully. If you are told you are not in the best of shape, don't let despondency discourage you. It probably means you have let your body down one way or another and only you can put it right.
3 So start where commonsense tells you to. Begin with the very basic breathing exercises (shown on p 86) and perhaps choose walking or swimming rather than strenuous effort like running or jogging.

CHECK BEFORE YOU BEGIN

POPULAR EXERCISES IN SUMMARY: WHAT'S BEST FOR ME?

ACTIVITY	INJURIES AND PRECAUTIONS	BENEFITS
Swimming	Swimmer's shoulders. Goggles are advisable to protect eyes.	Suitable for all ages. Excellent for entire body. You work against water, not body-weight. Firms and tones thighs and breasts/chest.
Running Jogging	Working against gravity. Harmful to spine. Shin splints, bone spurs, stress fractures, heat exhaustion. Painful kneecaps, due to knee stress, and surrounding tissues from pounding effect of running.	Efficient kilojoule burner. Works legs and thighs. Excellent for those with no anatomical disorders. Regular running improves wellbeing. Helps reduce weight.
Brisk Walking	Very few. Watch traffic and potholes. Avoid midday heat. Wear sensible flat shoes.	Walking is free! Increases metabolism, aids digestion. Good for all ages and everyone. Best all-round exercise for even the elderly.
Yoga	Overstretching is common. Knee injuries and neck injuries can occur if exercises are not done with experienced supervision.	Not suitable for those with unstab joints, high blood pressure, slippe disc, enlarged liver or spleen. Avo pressure on neck (Shoulder or Hea Stand, Plough, Karna Peedasana — choking pose).
Lifting Weights	Back injuries, joint strains, muscle tears. Not for people with heart problems or high blood pressure.	Can greatly improve shape. Increases overall metabolic rate.
Aerobic Dance	If done on thin carpet covering cement — groin pain, shin splints. Back pain, muscle strains. Orthopaedic injuries in lower extremities.	Total fitness as well as toning up bottom, thighs and stomach. Burns fat. Increases heart rate, improves cardiovascular system.
Tennis	Tennis elbow. Leg, ankle and knee injuries from sudden fast turns. Shoulder strains.	Good leg and upper arm firmer. Not for really overweight people with joint problems.
Bicycling	Some knee injuries and stress to lower back and neck. Stick to designated bike paths or the park.	Good all-round activity for heart/legs. Cardiovascular improvement. Firms legs, thighs and bottom.

FLEXIBILITY	MUSCLE STRENGTH	CARDIO-RESPIRATORY ENDURANCE	APPROXIMATE KJ PER HOUR
Yes	Will strengthen and firm quickly. Tones all muscles. Excellent for upper body and leg strength.	Good	Backstroke — 1800 Breaststroke — 1425 Crawl (Freestyle) — 2130
None. It is essential to warm-up and do some stretching exercises before and after.	Will not specifically improve upper body.	Excellent	Jogging at about 8 km/h — 1900–2514
None	Strengthens legs and thighs if you stride vigorously.	Excellent	Up stairs 4525 Down stairs 545 Uphill 1508 Flat at 5.5 km/hour 1100–1900
Excellent	Tones and firms	Not much	900
Nil Needs supplementing.	Excellent	Elevates heart rate and sustains it for 30 minutes.	2100
Stretching needed for body flexibility to avoid muscle injury.	Tones and firms	Improves cardiovascular system allowing the body more oxygen and better circulation.	Low-impact: Moderate — 880 Vigorous — 1341–1600 High impact — 1000
Nil	Yes	Good if done vigorously.	1700–1900 (singles)
Nil	Yes. Tones legs in particular.	Excellent	920–1400

WHAT EXERCISE EQUIPMENT WOULD SUIT YOUR NEEDS MOST?

EQUIPMENT	INJURIES	BENEFITS	DISADVANTAGES
Exercise Bike	Unlikely you'll fall off and hurt yourself. If you set the hill level too high, there could be tremendous pressure on the knees after a while.	Increases cardiovascular capacity. Firms and strengthens legs and buttocks. Can be used to warm up and cool down.	Must use for 15–20 minutes minimum. Can get boring. Equipment takes up space.
Treadmill	Can cause joint soreness.	Can be used indoors in cold or wet weather. Good for cardiovascular system. Firms legs.	Can get boring.
Rowing Machine	Motivation is the main problem as you need to increase speed once you reach your desired level.	Fitness. Strengthens upper body. Good aerobic exercise.	Resistance on some machines not adjustable. Not cheap. Space problem.
Skipping Rope	Possible joint injuries or muscle jarring.	Highly effective aerobic activity. Very cost efficient.	Can get boring. You need good shoes. Avoid concrete floors.

MAKING A START

This should be looked at with as much pleasure and optimism as you can muster. It is entirely true to say, 'The first few weeks are the hardest ...'; they really are. Once begun though, you will never look back and within, say, six weeks, you will truly wonder how you ever got by without it. Remind yourself of the basic preparation:

♦ Try to pick the time of day best suited to your lifestyle and stick to it. Don't do anything that you do not feel in harmony with. What is suited to someone else may be completely wrong for you.

♦ Always do less than you think you can in the early stages. Don't be overambitious. Remember, it took a long time to get into the condition you're in and it can't be corrected overnight. A slow methodical build-up is the only way to reach your personal goal and avoid disappointment in your performance and progress.

- Wear the right shoes and loose-fitting gear (there are many excellent brands to choose from). *Particularly important if you decide to run:* worn sneakers on roads or other hard surfaces are a formula for joint and back problems.
- Don't ever attempt back bends or waist exercises without adequate warm-up. Each forward bend toe touch places an average of 2757 kPa (28 kilograms per square centimetre) of pressure on your back. Countless weekend athletes sustain debilitating back injuries because of skipping the warm-up process. Nothing will stop your progress faster or surer than a pulled back muscle. Running puts 3447 kPa (35 kilograms per square centimetre) of pressure on each foot with every step taken. It's easy to see why, without proper stretching, it is asking for trouble.

THE IMPORTANCE OF FLEXIBILITY

We have already mentioned the importance of stretching exercises; here are some practical details. To the Chi Kung student as well as any serious athlete the practice of concentrated stretching before, during and after training is as automatic as getting out of bed. Anyone intending to exercise soon discovers the same, if not through instruction then through the pain and discomfort of a torn muscle or pulled ligament. It is an almost certain price for beginning to exercise without a thorough stretching routine. You must warm up your muscles, or be sure of a debilitating strain.

When your body is thoroughly flexible, each movement takes less work. Flexibility has been found to help avoid injuries, allowing you to perform better at work and play, tiring less quickly. When a muscle works, it uses up energy. This energy comes from the chemical action between glucose (stored in the muscle) and oxygen from the blood. The chemical action forms lactic acid. As the lactic acid builds up, the muscle begins to feel tired. When the muscle rests, the acid is reconverted to glucose. In a flexible person, this accumulation of lactic acid is carried away faster.

Habitual exercise such as jogging and running does not put muscles through their full range of motion, so they tend to shorten and pull on the lower back, causing strain. Whatever your sport, no matter how fit you are, five minutes of stretches before and after your workout can make the difference between pleasure and pain, progress or sports injury.

So, do *not* begin your exercise programme by suddenly bending and stretching. The average person's muscles aren't warm enough to tolerate the strain, especially in beginners and older people. Cold muscles and joints can react to sudden exertion by tearing. The heart also must be given time to increase its pace gradually. Start with at least five to ten minutes walking, trampolining, running on the spot, callisthenics, any form of limbering and warming up of your body before exerting pressure on muscles, tendons and ligaments.

Some days you may feel tighter or stiffer, so always work at your own pace and within your own limits. Muscles which should be included in your stretching routine are the hamstring, the lower back muscles, the hip muscles and thigh muscles. Now for the stretches; here are a few tips:

1 Start with easy stretches and *gradually* increase tension.

2 Your breathing should be consciously slow and rhythmic.

3 *Never* bend your back during your stretch. Bend at the hips, keeping your lower back straight. The forty-eight small muscles in the lower back are thin, quite delicate sheets and are most susceptible to tears.

4 Work slowly. Let the increased blood supply from stretching and relaxing work with you. Slow gentle movements, not to the point of pain, and hold for at least fifteen to twenty seconds. *Do not over-stretch.* Stretching too far can activate the stretch reflex, tightening the muscle you are trying to loosen.

5 *Do not bounce.* Avoid fast, bouncy, jerking motions. Concentrate on exercising slowly and smoothly. Your muscles will contract instead of relax when stretched forcibly. This can cause strain and tiny tears in the muscle fibre. When a muscle is stretched to its limit, a nervous connection to the brain (*golgi* reflex) causes the muscle to contract. If you bounce, it 'confuses' unconditioned muscle fibres as to which way to respond and can result in injury.

6 Work your muscles till you feel the tension. If you don't feel anything, it isn't making progress. You might have to hold a position longer, say up to thirty seconds.

7 If you are really stiff, a hot shower before a workout may do you more good than having one afterwards.

8 Pain is the body's signal to stop. Don't 'work through' pain, usually the result of a torn fibre in muscle, tendon or ligament. This will only hinder the healing process and encourage a more severe injury.

9 Don't eat a big meal within two to three hours of strenuous exercise, especially protein-high foods, as protein takes longer to digest than carbohydrates.

10 Cooling down after a workout is also most important. Allow at least five to ten minutes. Stopping suddenly after vigorous exercise can cause blood pressure to plummet and you may feel dizzy as the legs are no longer pushing blood to the heart. Stretching *after* a workout also prevents or at least reduces soreness, the following day.

Worth repeating. The thing to remember is that when sitting for long hours — as, say, in any desk-bound job — the back ligaments are continually stretched, which weakens the muscles. Prolonged standing — as with shop assistants — leads to the opposite: stiff compressed joints.

Muscles lose flexibility without regular stretching, then, when called upon to make any quick movement, this will cause a strain, or worse, a tear. So, regular stretching will help to:

♦ Increase stamina; because of increased blood supply and oxygen to the muscles.

♦ Reduce muscle tension, making you feel looser all over and therefore more relaxed.

♦ Prevent traumatic injuries.

♦ Increase your ability to relax physically and mentally.

♦ Promote better performance in work and play.

BASIC STRETCHES

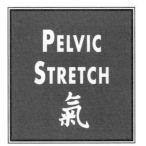

PELVIC STRETCH 氣

BENEFITS This exercise stretches out the upper and lower abdominals as well as the back. It strengthens the legs and back and improves spinal flexibility and elasticity. It also brings blood to the thyroids.

CAUTION Do not lift the hips too high off the floor because it puts pressure on your neck. This exercise is not suitable for those suffering high blood pressure or neck displacement.

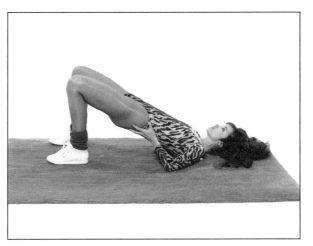

STEP 1 ▲

Lie on your back with knees bent, feet slightly apart. Support your lower back with your hands and raise your bottom off the floor. Hold for the count of six and then lower your back to the floor. Repeat 6 times.

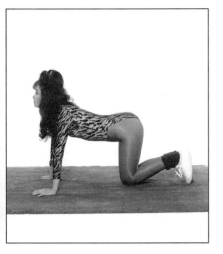 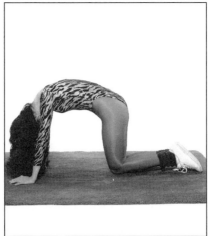

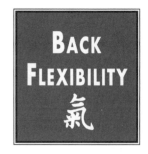

STEP 1 ▲

Position yourself on hands and knees with your hands about 30 to 33 centimetres apart, palms flat on the floor. Keep your arms straight. Breathe in, tilt your head back. Hollow your back in a concave line. Hold for the count of four.

STEP 2 ▲

Breathe out, arch your back, raise it to a hump. Hold for the count of four.

BENEFITS This stretch brings flexibility to your spine and is a safe exercise for all ages. It helps relieve lower back ache and tension. In time, the arms and shoulders will also be strengthened. This is an ideal antenatal and postnatal exercise.

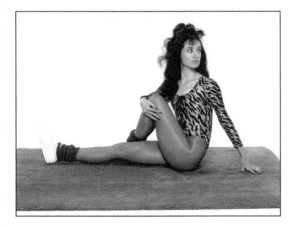

◄ **STEP 1**

Sit up straight on the floor, right leg outstretched in front. Bend your left knee and cross your left foot over to rest on the outside of your right knee. Press the left hip to the floor. The right arm goes across your upper left thigh. Look over your left shoulder.

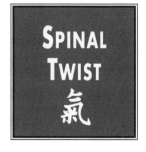

SPINAL TWIST 氣

BENEFITS This exercise forces energy up the spine and is good for the nervous system. It also stretches the outer thigh.

ACHILLES, CALF AND HAMSTRING STRETCH

氣

CAUTION Do not round your back in these exercises. The object is to get your chest to your thighs, not your nose to your knee. Do not stretch beyond the point where you begin to feel tension. Don't bounce or jerk.

STEP 1 ▶

Sit on the floor, legs straight out in front. Place your right heel on top of your left toe. Pull your chest down. Hold the stretch. Do the same with the other leg.

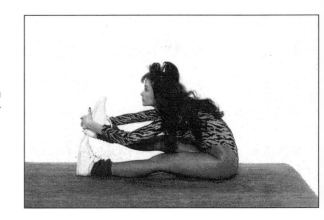

STEP 2 ▶

Sit on the floor, legs straight out in front. Cross your legs at the ankles and pull your chest forward. Hold the position. Do the same with the other leg on the top.

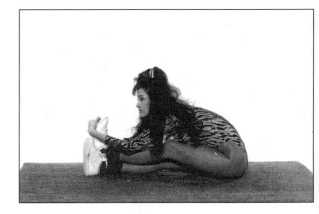

STEP 3 ▶

Sit on the floor, both legs together and straight out in front. Reach over and hold your ankles or toes. Hold the stretch.

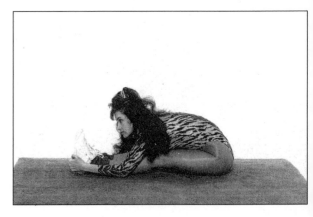

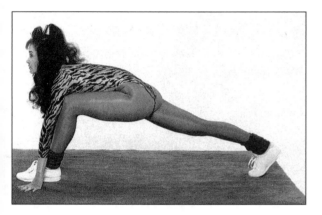

◄ **STEP 1**

Lunge forward keeping your back leg straight. Your front thigh should be parallel to the floor. Hold for the count of six. Repeat using the other leg.

CAUTION The front bent knee has to be in line with the front foot. Do not push your front knee too far forward because this will put too much pressure on the knee.

STEP 2 ►

Lunge forward keeping the back leg straight. Flex the foot of the straight leg and bring it towards your bottom. Put your weight on the thigh, not the kneecap. Hold for the count of four. Repeat using the other leg.

CAUTION The front knee must remain in line with the front foot. Do not put weight on the kneecap when you bend the back leg.

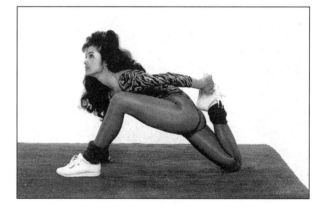

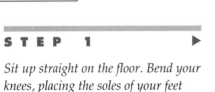

GROIN STRETCH 氣

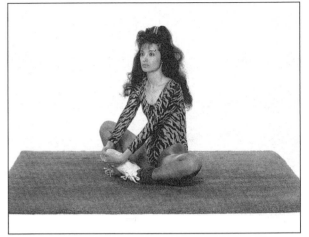

STEP 1 ▶

Sit up straight on the floor. Bend your knees, placing the soles of your feet together. Hold your ankles.

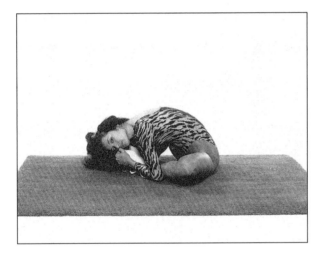

◀ STEP 2

Push your knees down with your elbows. Slowly and gently pull your upper body forwards keeping a straight back. Hold for the count of eight and gradually increase to sixteen.

CAUTION Bend from your hips. Do not round your back. Stop at the point of discomfort. Do not force yourself. This exercise stretches the adductors (inner thigh muscles) which give your knees their stability. It is important not to force this stretch as the adductors are easily pulled and take time to heal.

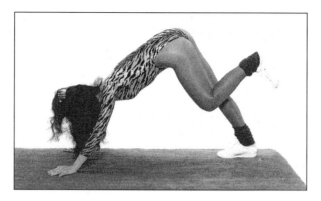

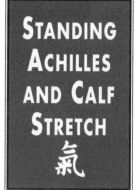

STANDING ACHILLES AND CALF STRETCH 氣

STEP 1 ▲

Stand with your palms on the floor in front of your body. Walk the hands forward away from your body. Keep one leg straight with the heel on the floor. Alternate legs four times.

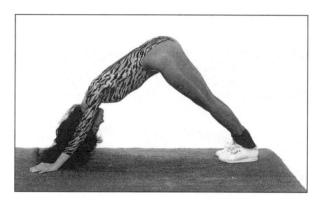

STEP 2 ▶

Finally, try to get both heels down on the floor and hold for the count of six.

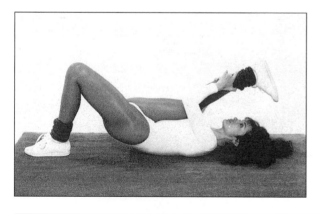

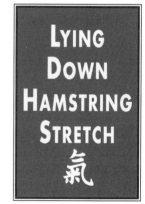

LYING DOWN HAMSTRING STRETCH 氣

STEP 1 ▲

Lie on the floor and bend your knees, keeping your feet flat on the floor. Bring your right knee towards your chest and wrap your arm around your knee. Slip your hands underneath the right thigh and straighten your leg, flexing the foot. Hold for the count of six. Lower your right leg and repeat on the left side.

If you are flexible, extend your lower leg instead of keeping it bent.

LYING DOWN ABDUCTOR STRETCH
氣

BENEFITS This is particularly good for stretching overworked muscles after you have been doing a lot of side leg lifts or raises.

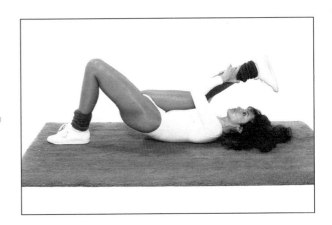

STEP 1 ▶

Lie on your back, bend both knees keeping your feet flat on the floor. Bring the right knee towards your chest (as in the hamstring stretch).

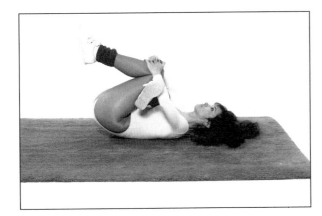

◀ STEP 2

Lift your left leg across your right leg. Wrap your arm around the left knee. Hug it as close to your chest as you can. Hold for the count of six. You should now feel the stretch on the outside of your left thigh.

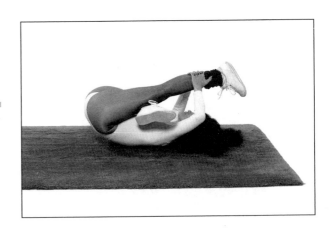

STEP 3 ▶

If you are flexible, extend the left leg. Slip your hands around the back of the left leg and bring it as close to your chest as possible. Hold for the count of six.

ADVANCED STRETCHES

STEP 1 ▶

Start with your hands on the floor, legs apart and both straight.

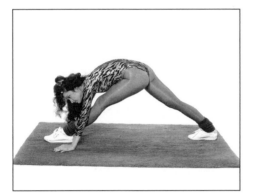

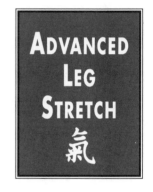

ADVANCED LEG STRETCH

◀ **STEP 2**

Lower yourself onto your right leg, slide your left leg forwards keeping your left leg straight with toes pointed up.

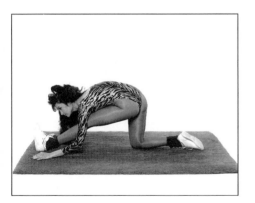

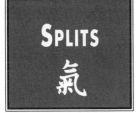

SPLITS

氣

BENEFITS This exercise stretches the legs, inner thighs and hip areas. The lower back and abdominal muscles are also loosened.

CAUTION Only attempt the split when maximum flexibility has been achieved through practising the advanced leg stretch. The splits should be tried slowly and with extreme care to avoid strain. Only attempt it if you are already extremely flexible in the groin and leg muscles.

S T E P   1   ▶

Start with the advanced leg stretch (you can do it with either leg forwards), then lower your chest to your leg.

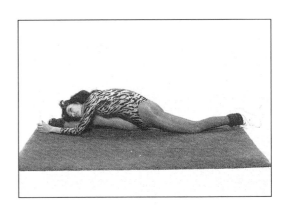

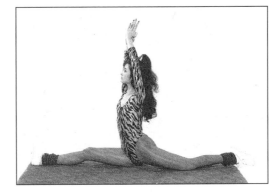

◀   S T E P   2

Straighten up slowly, stretching your abdominal muscles.

BENEFITS It stretches the hips, inner thighs and groin muscles. When the upper body is angled forward, the lower back is stretched as well.

CAUTION Attempt this exercise only when properly warmed up. This is a very advanced exercise and provides a radical stretch to the leg muscles. Patience is necessary. Expect slow results.

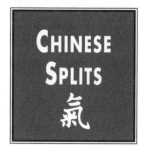

CHINESE SPLITS
氣

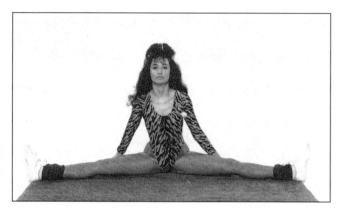

◀ **S T E P 1**

Sit with your legs as wide apart as you can manage.

S T E P 2 ▶

Pull your chest close to your right thigh. Hold it for eight counts. Then take it to your left thigh and hold it for eight counts.

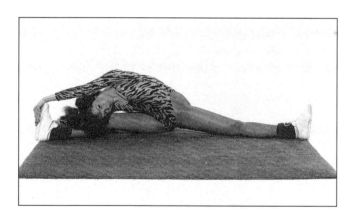

◀ **S T E P 3**

Pull your body to the centre and lower your chest forward as far as you can. Don't force or strain. Hold for eight counts.

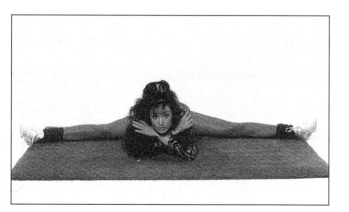

WALKING — THE BEST ACTIVITY

Walking is the best activity for the most dedicated exercise hater and the most natural of all. Regular walking can be just as rewarding, more enjoyable and free of the prospect of the short- or long-term injury that sometimes goes with jogging. It is non-competitive, without the pressure of success or failure, progress or the lack of it. You can walk any time and anywhere and if you are not an exhibitionist like the dedicated city runner intent on being seen, you won't get noticed. It is also an excellent opportunity to practise breathing, teach yourself breath control and improve your lung capacity. Like Chi Kung, it needs no special clothing, apparatus, training facility or partner.

Walking is an excellent way of measuring and increasing your inhalations and exhalations. Sometimes called yogic walking, it is said to have been used by yogis on their often endless pilgrimages across India.

Start by breathing in slowly and steadily (through the nose) and count how many paces it takes to breathe in, how many paces you can hold it for, and how many paces it takes to breathe out.

If you are a fairly normal breather and walk at a normal pace, you'll probably find it takes say three paces to breathe in, you can hold it for three, and breathe out for three. The out-breath may be longer than the in-breath. (*Kumbaka*, the yogic word for breath holding, is not suitable for pregnant women.)

Practise doing this, always remembering to concentrate on the lower Tan T'ien and breathing accordingly, and gradually increase the number of paces, not by speeding up but by keeping your normal pace and lengthening your inhalation, holding capacity and exhalation.

If you walk regularly and remember to practise yogic breathing, you'll find that three paces will soon become four, then five, six and so on until you reach around twelve paces to breathe in, twelve paces to hold and twelve paces to breathe out. By that time your lung capacity and breath control will have increased and you will be far better equipped for Chi Kung.

Walking is particularly valuable if you are on a diet. Like most forms of moderate exercise, it works to tone up internal stomach and digestive tract muscles, which tends to decrease appetite. If under stress, or bored, a good walk in the fresh air is a far better remedy than reaching for the biscuits or that pastry you've been saving for an emergency. By the time you get back, you won't need it.

Walking also improves muscle conditioning without actually building up muscles the way weight-training does. It streamlines and tones up the body without unwanted changes in shape.

Even your posture improves with walking. You move, sit or stand more gracefully. When you begin to feel better through regular walks, increasing distance and pace, you look better, feel more confident and improve your all-round performance.

Walking helps reduce stress for although it is a very definite form of exercise when pursued with energy, it is also an extremely effective method of relaxation. When walking, the body is largely switched over to a motor reflex which needs no concentration, leaving the mind to unwind and sort out its problems — unfolding with the changing scenery. So walking may give greater benefit than more exacting activities that require undivided attention and coordination.

Another big plus for walkers is that it is entirely safe to practise, with very little danger of any form of strain through overexertion.

Walking is subject to no age limit or fitness level. It is ideal for recuperation from illness, hospitalisation or surgery, when the body has been forced to rest and needs to be reactivated. It provides a gentle workout that can be stepped up as vigour and energy return.

An excellent break from the office or any enclosed environment when the head needs clearing, even a turn around the block can change perspective and stimulate ideas, especially when supplemented by deep breathing. The rules are simple but important:

♦ Wear comfortable shoes.
♦ As with most exercise, don't go at it like a bull at a gate. Start at a leisurely pace and increase distance and speed as you go but break through the strolling or sauntering stage as soon as you can.
♦ If you are not used to walking and distance daunts you, don't be overambitious. Set your target and stick to it, lengthen it as you go, say half a kilometre at a time. Stick to flat areas, leaving the hills till later.
♦ You can use walking to expand your senses — enjoy early dewy mornings at sunrise, the beauty of a sunset or a full moon or a starry sky — the choice is yours.
♦ Never look at walking as a waste of time. Medical scientists are fast realising that it is one of the safest, surest, most natural health benefits we can pursue.

CHI KUNG
AND AGEING

Of the many benefits attributed to breath therapy the preservation of youthfulness has always been considered an art. It does not mean that all Orientals live longer and healthier lives than we in the West. Although the Asian approach to preventive medicine and a lower consumption of fat may reduce the risk of some ageing diseases for the man and woman in the street, it is those that practise Chi Kung who remain alert, agile and strong into old age.

By 'gracefully', the Chinese do not necessarily mean cosmetically. The principles of Chinese physical culture seldom consider the outward appearance above the internal condition. Some of the most powerful exponents of Chi Kung or Kung Fu are physically insignificant men and women, often with very little obvious muscular development. Those that reach the level of master are usually over the age of forty or fifty and continue developing their powers and teaching their skills well into their eighties and beyond, many living active lives as Sifus (teachers) to well over one hundred.

This says much for the rejuvenating effects of Chi Kung upon organs that would certainly degenerate without the restorative stimulation and internal massaging of Chi Kung with its constant refreshing and energising of the blood. Breathing exercises are also greatly favoured by the elderly because one is never too old to learn, they are not too strenuous, once a set of exercises has been learned they can be practised privately, they are non-competitive and natural in every way, without the need of anything but one's own concentration on the patient persuasion of the body. The elderly are also more likely to achieve the state of quietude essential to effective Chi Kung and have more time to practise a regular routine with the necessary diligence.

The introductory breathing exercises shown on pages 86–90 are ideal for the older person. Even if taken no further they will at least improve breathing habits. Depending upon the individual condition and degree of determination, they can gradually pave the way for the slightly more advanced forms of exercise that call for increased physical activity and the improvement of lost flexibility. If the introductory exercises — lying, sitting, standing — are taken further, the warning of patience and tolerance in making progress is especially important to those of middle age and older, particularly those in poor health, suffering from any illness or disability or recovering from injury.

Chi Kung alone, however, cannot guarantee a worthwhile improvement unless other aspects of the ageing process are understood and attended to. The Chinese preoccupation with staying young and living as long as possible is reflected in the food they eat, the liquids they drink and the medicines they take. Great credibility (and often very large amounts of money) is given to the restorative properties of foods, drinks and herbal mixtures that stimulate vitality and promote longevity.

The maximum human life span seems to be around 120 years. A considerable number of people have been known to reach this incredible age. There have even been stories of some who lived beyond this age in both China and India with one, a Chinese philosopher and master of Chi Kung, who is said to have lived to 202 years of age. His photograph, taken by one of Shanghai's first photographers on the old master's two hundredth birthday, has found its way into many books on Kung Fu. Most reports of extreme longevity reach us from the East and almost always of those living simple and very natural lifestyles, often in high mountainous regions where air is at its best, soil remains purely organic and the effects of modern progress are minimal.

The advances of modern medicine and public health since the turn of the century have lifted the average life expectancy from fifty to seventy-five years. With the growing interest in healthier lifestyles, a new awareness of alternate methods of exercise, relaxation and nutrition, it is possible that the average life expectancy will reach eighty-five years within the foreseeable future.

There is, of course, a condition to this new-found promise of long life. Unless we really work at it and make the effort to help ourselves, three out of four extra years gained will be burdened with the degenerative process of ageing that until now has been accepted as unavoidable: loss of strength and coordination; arthritic complaints; respiratory and heart conditions; the failing of sight, hearing and memory; hypertension and blood pressure; and, of course, increased vulnerability to injury and diseases such as Alzheimers and Parkinsons. If the body's resistance isn't kept up and the immune system regularly fortified the ability to heal ourselves will disappear altogether with advancing years.

HOW AND WHEN DO WE BEGIN TO GROW OLD?

In a society all but overwhelmed by the youth cult, where ageing is at best not contemplated and barely tolerated, it is interesting to know that we begin to grow old in our twenties. In the United States, the government is spending US$2 billion on gerontological research — the study of ageing. Their findings show that at birth we come complete with a built-in obsolescence already programmed into our genes. In our twenties, our skin begins to dry out and become increasingly susceptible to blemishes. Unless it is properly cared for it will become wrinkled and blotchy by the time we reach fifty and rapidly deteriorate from there.

At twenty-five our metabolism is already showing signs of slowing down and we need fewer kilojoules to maintain our body-weight. As we age, substances such as cholesterol and calcium tend to become stored in body cells instead of dissolving and passing through the digestive system as efficiently as they should, so diet also becomes more and more important as we grow older.

Between the ages of thirty and seventy we lose 30 to 40 per cent of our muscle if we don't exercise it on a continual basis. Regular aerobic exercise and careful stretching can reverse this deterioration up to twenty years.

Around the age of thirty our immune system begins to weaken. The vital thymus gland responsible for the rapid reproduction of white blood cells, our main defence against disease, is one of the first to slow down. The less we do to rejuvenate it, the faster it will give up and the more vulnerable we will become.

Most of our other vital organs begin to suffer the onslaught of age after thirty. Our kidneys can lose up to 50 per cent of their function, lungs 30 to 50 percent of their capacity for taking in air (particularly if we smoke) and much of our liver function will have been destroyed depending on how much we may have abused it in the first half of our lives.

At forty, vision will almost certainly begin to lose its sharpness and around sixty we may be troubled with cataracts unless the practice of eye exercises prevents it. Also around forty women will begin to lose bone because of an inability to properly absorb calcium, an ageing condition that can also be improved through the right amount of exercise along with supplementary diet.

By the time we reach sixty, brain shrinkage may begin to affect our recall and memory performance. Unless we see to it that our minds are kept active, loss of memory becomes a sort of self-fulfilling prophecy. We may activate the program of old age by convincing ourselves that we are wearing out our minds and bodies and are therefore of no further use to ourselves, those around us or the world. Mental stimulation of any sort will help prevent this process indefinitely.

Inevitable as ageing appears to be, it need not be as gloomy as it sometimes sounds. Staying young can become a project that is both enjoyable, fulfilling and extremely rewarding.

If there is a 'fountain of youth' we haven't found it yet and must content ourselves with commonsense ways to stay younger than our calendar years until someone comes along with a miracle cure. In the meantime, most medical researchers agree on a fairly predictable and often repeated set of principles:

COMMON- SENSE WAYS TO STAY YOUNG

♦ Change your diet to avoid foods over rich in cholesterol and saturated fats — eggs, beef, butter, lard, too many dairy foods (especially ice cream), bacon, and other delicatessen temptations. Replace them with skinless chicken or turkey, fish (not shellfish), any of the plentiful high fibre cereals and wholegrain breads available. Learn about and plan high nutrition, low-kilojoule diet programs of your own choosing.

You don't have to deprive yourself of everything you like but learn to balance your diet and supplement those vitamins and minerals modern foods are deficient in. Grow your own herbs and shoots. (Wheatgrass juice, for example, is a great blood cleanser — it can be bought cheaply from any health store. It is easy to grow and is ready to cut in 3 to 4 days. Its juice is amazingly refreshing and has exceptional healing qualities). If you're lucky enough to have the space to grow your own vegetables and fruit, get back to nature with real organic gardening and you'll gain from the nutrition and from the exercise. Remember the old masters and their theory of Yin and Yang.

♦ Stay out of the midday sun. Limited sunshine to the body early or late in the day when its rays are less damaging can be good for you but too much, too hot is asking for trouble.

♦ Drink plenty of water. Many of us overlook the cleansing effect of clean, clear water. We have spent a lifetime drinking everything else, tea, coffee, soft drinks, wines, spirits and beer — all of which contain water. Maybe it's time to start drinking it neat, just plain, fresh water first thing in the morning and last thing at night. If you consider a purifier, make sure you choose a reliable brand — water filtering systems can be expensive and ineffectual.

♦ Cut back on alcohol if you can't give it up altogether. More and more medical researchers are, however, suggesting that a couple of beers a day can be beneficial, especially the dark ale or stout variety. Guinness in particular contains iron as well as other nutrients which outweigh the adverse effect of alcohol if enjoyed in moderation.

♦ Do all that you can to achieve a cut down on medication. A large majority of people over sixty-five (and many much younger) have allowed themselves to become overmedicated. Nearly 80 per cent are reliant on medication for at least one chronic condition — arthritis, heart, blood pressure, hearing failure or other degenerative diseases. Around 30 per cent of those may have three or more such ailments to combat with as many as five different prescriptions. Overmedication of this kind can cause mental confusion, impaired circulation and blood clotting, which in turn can cause cardiac disturbance and joint problems. Closer attention to self-help through more natural remedies can slowly diminish the need for some synthetic drugs.

♦ Stop smoking. Too much has already been said about the dangers of smoking and there isn't a smoker today who isn't well aware of the possible consequences. They also know that the various methods of stopping, for example, hypnotherapy and acupuncture, will not work without good old-fashioned willpower. Breathing exercises can be an immense help in overcoming the nervous tension or sheer habit of smoking. After a few weeks of concentrated breathing exercises the craving for tobacco is replaced by the pleasure of breathing freely and fully. Within a period of four to six weeks the need will have been replaced permanently.

♦ Reduce negative stress which will eventually lead to anxiety and depression. The adverse effects of stress can be reduced by limiting the unenjoyable tasks of everyday living. It isn't easy but it can be done. Think twice about becoming involved in things or with people you really do not like. Is it essential? Can it wait? Can it be avoided altogether? Often it can and should be replaced with something you do enjoy. Depression can be mistaken for senility or dementia in the elderly. It is a much ignored disorder that we can do something to fight no matter what its causes. Methods of relaxation (of which breathing exercises can be a very important part) and deep contemplation of the more pleasurable aspects of life leading to simple forms of meditation will help avoid the anxiety states that can trigger depression, or help you break out of black moods.

♦ Exercise at least twenty to thirty minutes no less than three times a week. This is the bare minimum of exercise your body needs to keep bones strong, maintain or build muscle strength and flexibility, condition the heart and lungs, keep the circulation moving, the veins and arteries open and the Ch'i channels clear. The more you exercise the better you will feel and the longer you will enjoy being alive.

♦ Finally, don't let yourself be talked into growing old. Your biological age is not determined by your calendar age. In other words the number of birthdays you have seen come and go do not have to relate directly to how old you are unless you let them. Nothing is more open to negative and positive thought than the question of age. Dr Charles Champton of the University of Miami Medical School sums it up very well.

Your actual (calendar) age may be 40 but the biological age of your heart may be 50, your muscles and ligaments 60, your lungs, liver, kidneys and other vital organs 65 and your brain three-score and ten.

On the other hand, your calendar age may be 75 but the biological age of your heart may be 47, your muscles and ligaments 50, your vital organs 55 and your brain somewhere in-between.

NUTRITION AND THE POWER OF CH'I

PART TEN

THE CHINESE ATTITUDE TO NUTRITION AND CHI KUNG

To the Chinese Masters of yesterday and the fitness enthusiast of today the choosing and matching of food is as essential to the vital balance of health as is the science of breath. But finding and eating just the right food in just the right quantities at just the right times has become difficult to do as progress takes the place of tradition, quantity outweighs quality and expediency overtakes authenticity in the producing, preparing and eating of food. In spite of the improvements in food technology over the past decade, selection of the right foods has become even more confusing.

The Oriental attitude to nutrition is also very little different from ours, with one important difference. There are two main reasons for pursuing an individual diet, consideration of one's health in the interests of a long, enjoyable life, and concern for one's appearance in the interests of vanity and an eventful sex life. The Oriental is interested more in the first, the average Westerner is likely to be more interested in the second. The crash diet in all its wondrous forms is as yet virtually unknown in Asia but has become a conventional part of life in most Western societies.

As children, we tend to overindulge in whatever foods take our fancy — if we are allowed to — but with little or no ill effect because we burn up whatever we eat with boundless energy.

Disregard for our eating habits and their long-term effects continues through the teenage spin of fast food, soft drink and confectionery into adulthood — where it is often supplemented with alcohol and tobacco — until for one reason or another, often the opinion of someone of the opposite sex, we realise that we are getting fat and unhealthy, our complexion may not be as clear as we would like and the flow of energy we have relied upon to propel us uninterrupted through life is beginning to let us down.

An awareness of responsibility towards our one and only body, which can range from cautious questioning to outright panic, presents itself if we are sensible enough to recognise its cry for help. The seesawing between programs of disciplined eating and periods of gorging only serves to confuse the body further.

Even if we maintain a strict diet — and few of us do — this does not necessarily mean that the romantic side of life will vastly improve or the promotion that we have hoped for will suddenly be ours.

Worse than this, we may be feeding one set of glands or organs while starving another, unsettling a digestive and absorption system that has become thoroughly accustomed to coping with the eating habits of a lifetime as best it can. Imbalance is the thing the Chinese attitude to food and health tries hardest to avoid, believing that certain foods and flavours together with correct breathing and moderate exercise is the key to long life, mental and emotional stability and even material prosperity.

This does not mean that every Oriental adheres strictly to the enlightened dietary opinions of his or her ancestors. You only have to explore a Chinese grocery store to become lost in the world of exotic foodstuffs that break all the rules — an endless array of canned and bottled delicacies, some of which exceed the wildest imagination, all spiced, pickled and preserved together with a multitude of sauces and condiments far removed from the Taoist concept of natural nourishment.

In the East as in the West there is a marked difference between the dietary health of the city dweller and the person who lives and works in the country. The peasant has some distinct advantages over those brought up in the city — plainer, more natural and usually fresher food, cleaner air and purer water and regular exercise through physical labour. Whether it is a farming or fishing family of rural Europe, Southeast Asia or country Australia, they are likely to live longer, work harder and maintain good health longer than those in the city exposed to a wider variety of convenience foods and the air and water treatments massed communities create or require.

Before going further, it will be helpful if we consider that often seen but too little understood Chinese symbol of the balance of negative and positive, light and darkness, masculine and feminine principles — the Yin and the Yang.

As Chinese medicine becomes more accessible to the ordinary people of Western countries, so interest in the philosophies and beliefs behind it grow. Until perhaps a decade ago that interest was shown by a very small group of enthusiasts, dabblers or serious students, often connected with Oriental martial arts.

Throughout Europe, America and Australia the various forms of Kung Fu, Tai Chi Tuan, Karate and Tae Kwan Do are being taught by Asian Masters and those select Western adepts who, generally having been taught by Oriental experts, have withstood the demands and disciplines expected of them, endured and triumphed over years of arduous training and emerged as instructors or Masters with or without the blessings of their patient teachers.

This is nothing new. Wherever the Asian Master settles, his/her style or form of self-defence goes too, and with it his/her philosophy, knowledge of training methods, preventive medicine and healing. This has been the case for centuries, but the phenomenon of the Western student is comparatively new. Today, Westerners of all ages and types and both sexes, are seeking out self-improvement regimes of the ancient East.

Among the mysteries that the non-Asian must come to grips with is the concept of Yin and Yang — that mystic balance upon which all things in Chinese medicine depend. The Yin–Yang symbol of light and dark, the passive and the aggressive, symbolic embryo of sickness and health, of life and death — curl around each other in perfect harmony, taking up identical space in the circle of the universe, keeping the delicate balance of life.

It is maintaining this vital balance at all times that the Chinese believe is the secret of health and wellbeing. In its simplest form we can see that if we become too hot (what the Chinese call 'fiery' or 'heatiness' and what we call 'feverish'), we become redder, darker, the skin more suffused with blood. Then we are overly Yang — the Yang is overpowering the Yin. A Yang person is likely to be hyperactive, more prone to hypertensive tendencies and high blood pressure, possibly heart trouble.

If we become too cold (what the Chinese call 'foong' or 'windiness' and we call damp or wet) we become paler, weaker, less energetic. Then we are overly Yin — the Yin is overpowering the Yang. A Yin person is likely to be lethargic, more prone to anaemia, lack of energy and open to infection.

YIN AND YANG — THE TAO: CENTRE OF BALANCE

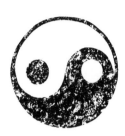

The Yin-Yang symbol

The Taoist sages claimed that the first god of medicine, long before the Yellow Emperor and in the very beginning, was Pan Ku. After the universe was rent with what some consider as the Big Bang, Pan Ku started to pick up the pieces. In order to make some kind of sense of

WHERE DID IT ALL BEGIN?

what was left, he began by sorting things into an order which he called the Yin and the Yang.

Into the Yang he placed the masculine, the active, the brightness and warmth. Yang was the life-giver, the celestial body from which all power comes.

The Yin he set aside as the feminine, the dark, mysterious and cold. Yin was the inanimate, the emptiness which unless filled and illuminated by the Yang, becomes hollow and dead.

Perhaps the greatest exponent of Yin and Yang was China's greatest and most influential teacher and philosopher. Confucius-Kung-Fu-Tzu, about 511–479 BC. Orphaned early in life from a noble but impoverished family, Confucius' thirst for understanding set him on a path of self-education and seeking of truth that was to form the foundation of later Chinese culture.

He saw the compatible merging of Yin and Yang as the only true path to physical harmony and spiritual enlightenment and he called that path — the 'Tao', the Way. Whatever interfered with the Tao, the essential balance, was to be avoided at all costs.

Another famous Chinese thinker of the sixth century BC was the wise and venerable Lao Tzu, who held that the practice of moderation, humility and morality was the key to health and longevity, an attitude that is surely as valid today as it was then. Overeating and overdrinking, the push for power or money and the pursuit of indiscriminate sex certainly isn't doing us any good.

Refusal to recognise the Tao, to ignore the Way and take another path was to disobey the laws of nature and become undone. Besides this, however, were the facts of illness and injury caused by factors beyond our control. To avert these all too real possibilities Lao Tzu and those that followed him focused on prevention rather than cure, the essence of Taoism and still the basis of Chinese medicine today.

As to injury, well as we have learned, the pursuit of health and avoidance of illness through correct living and natural means extended to the discovery and nurturing of the life force and developed in turn into techniques of self-defence to minimise the danger of attack as well as absorb its effects.

These attitudes put China in the forefront of medical progress while Western civilisation was still suffering plague and pestilence unchecked. By the fourteenth century, Chinese midwives were practising obstetrics; the need for exercises, balanced diet, massage and breathing techniques were all recognised as well as specific treatments. The approach to healing was always an holistic* one — to

* 'Holistic' is a word coined by the famous South African general, Jan Christiaan Smuts. It asserts that the fundamental principle of the universe is the creation of wholes — complete and self-contained systems; complete forms of life and mind.

heal the spirit, treat the whole body, nourish and revitalise the internal organs and apply appropriate methods to put the patient back on the path — restore the Tao, balance the Yin and the Yang. Their methods, still essential to today's Chinese doctor, included acupuncture, heat application, bone setting and acupressure or deep tissue massage.

So through the Tao there evolved many bypaths of medicine and human conditioning. Tai Chi and Chi Kung were developed to keep fit and restore wellbeing. Diet became one of the essential means of restoring the equilibrium of Yin and Yang.

Natural nutrition was directly associated with the seasons and the five main elements that benefited the body: sour-tasting foods were believed to be good for the bones, pungent foods for the tendons, sweet for the muscles, salty for the blood and bitter for the lungs and throat.

No matter how obscure these beliefs may seem in today's synthetic existence, they are finding increasing acceptance by Western medical science. It does make sense to eat with the seasons, which means fruit, vegetables and grains in season rather than frozen, dried or preserved, which is exactly what nutritionists and naturopaths are telling us today. And aren't we constantly discovering the direct relationship between certain health complaints and particular foods?

Are not the greatest health hazards today the results of overindulgence in food, alcohol, tobacco and drugs? Isn't the rat-race resulting in an epidemic of stress — the *distress* that can lead to anything from a headache to malignant disease?

Shouldn't we then face up to the need to prevent illness rather than expect its cure; shouldn't we recognise the essential function of our organs and make some attempt to take care of them; accept the need for relaxation and look for ways to achieve periods of tranquility to help us cope?

So, Confucius and old Lao Tzu were right on the ball. There is a right and wrong way and there certainly is a correct balance between good and bad, right and wrong, black and white, Yin and Yang.

CH'ANG MING — TAOIST LONG LIFE

So, how did the Taoists of old, the hedgerow healers and 'barefoot doctors' of the past perceive nutrition and how does it relate today?

The principles of Ch'ang Ming are expressed in what is called the 'Six Prescriptions', based on the realisation that human beings come in different shapes and sizes and have totally different nutritional requirements. The folk healers recognised six distinct types based upon the Yang or positive person and the Yin or negative person. A Yang man for instance, is likely to be deep-chested, wide shouldered and slim-hipped; far more positive, strong and confident in mind and body than his slightly framed and more negative Yin counterpart. Likewise, a Yang woman will probably have a solid, more shapely form plus the outgoing personality that usually goes with it, while her Yin sister is slimmer, more delicate, less energetic and possibly less sure of herself in every way.

These two fundamental types are then subdivided further and their ideal diets prescribed accordingly:

1 *Heavy and positive* (**very Yang**): almost certain to have an efficient digestive system with excellent powers of absorption and distribution of nourishment. Should eat less high-calorie, energising foods and more raw fruit and vegetables.

2 *Heavy and negative* (**very Yin**): likely to have poor metabolism, weak digestion and sluggish absorption of nourishment. Would be prescribed foods that strengthen heart and liver function and advised to increase intake of water.

3 *Lean and positive* (**a little on the Yang side**): abounding in nervous energy and unlikely to gain unwanted weight, may be victim of an inefficient spleen, thin or toxic blood and poor circulation of Ch'i. Would be told to eat foods that promote the function of the spleen and strengthen the Ch'i to restore balance but do not overstimulate the heart or emotions.

4 *Lean and negative* (**a little on the Yin side**): weak internally, therefore fresh vegetables so suitable to the Yang constitution are too 'wet' for this system, laying it open to chills. Suggested that vegetables should always be steamed or lightly cooked and energising foods rich in calories be taken regularly to stimulate the Ch'i and restore balance of Yin and Yang.

5 *Nervous and positive* (**a lot on the Yang side**): also experiences poor circulation and inadequate digestion which can create a badly balanced nervous system swinging between hyperactivity and lethargy — always up and down. Such people would be strongly advised to avoid the overstimulation of too much caffeine (coffee) or tannin (tea) and certainly to cut down on processed, highly spiced foods containing preservatives and flavour additives such as delicatessen, frozen or take-away foods, and salt and monosodium glutamate.

6 *Nervous and negative* (**a lot on the Yin side**): a main problem with this type of constitution is inefficient elimination of waste and the tendency to store toxins. This in time begins to poison the system and impede the free flow of Ch'i, resulting in fatigue and if not corrected undermining the immune system. Would also be warned to stay away from overstimulating foods that contain artificial properties which the system cannot clear. Natural foods that help to build up liver, kidney and spleen activity would be prescribed.

All of these types would also be advised to improve respiration, cleanse the blood and stimulate the organs through breathing exercises.

The Six Prescriptions are related to the Five Flavours of Life: Bitter for the heart, Sour for the liver, Sweet for the spleen and colon, Pungent for the lungs and Salty for the kidneys. These in turn are related to particular grains, fruit and vegetables which again relate to the Four Seasons: Spring, Summer, Autumn and Winter, and the Five Elements: Wood, Fire, Earth, Metal and Water, which together make up the traditional Chinese way of comprehending the universe and the secrets of human existence.

This all sounds very confusing, particularly to the lover of Chinese food who regularly experiences the delights of Chinese cuisine, probably the most exotic and varied in the world. The fast, high-heat, stir-fry Cantonese cooking of Hong Kong; the hearty Chiu Chow food of Swatow and Guangdong washed down with bitter Iron Buddha tea; Pekinese dishes originating in the Imperial courts of emperors and empresses, highly flavoured with peppers, garlic, ginger, leek and coriander; the sweeter and oilier creations of Shanghai with their heavy, rich sauces, salted meats and pickled vegetables; the spicy, fiery delights of Szechuan hot and tasty with chilli and peppercorns.

Where are the principles of the Six Prescriptions in this delightful mix? Believe it or not the basics are always there: choice of food and style of cooking is designed to suit the province and its climate. Main ingredients are always market fresh, organically grown and never overcooked, vegetables always crisp and lightly done. Herbs, spices and other condiments are always natural — an artificial or synthetic additive would be unthinkable. (Mai Jing — monosodium glutamate, MSG — or the salt and pepper shakers are usually only found in restaurants) Meat is almost always lean and thinly cut, sliced or diced small so smaller amounts are consumed and the bulk of any dish is partly cooked vegetables and the staple rice or noodles. Fish and seafood abounds and the ever-present Ching Cha — green tea — or herb tea aids digestion.

To the Chinese, eating out is a way of life and the serious enjoyment of food is a regular ritual to those who can afford it. For those who cannot, meals are no less an occasion. The poorest coolies engaged in hard labour on Hong Kong or Chinese building sites will fortify themselves with a humble but highly nutritious dish of 'Jook' or rice conjee, a simple rice broth spiked with chives, containing chicken, meat or fish and a dash of sesame oil. The Tanks fisherman survives almost entirely on fish, rice and a little green vegetable. The Haaka woman will work her rice paddy from dawn to dusk on the simplest of meals — and fresh eggs — but all are relished as though they were a palace banquet.

DIET AND CHI KUNG

Even the master of Kung Fu or the teacher of Chi Kung would not argue with Confucius, who said 'Man cannot be too serious about his eating.' They accept the age-old Chinese concept that food is life, and is also health, strength, nourishment of the soul and a symbol of other good things such as luck, prosperity and (always) virility. 'Heaven loves a man who eats well', and each meal he enjoys adds to his virtue, strengthening his resistance to ills of body, mind and spirit, curing ailments and rendering him capable of better work and certainly better results. We are also, of course, eating to stay alive.

We choose our food for the tastes we prefer rather than for what the body needs; if the choices we make happen to fall into the right nutritional category, this is usually through luck rather than management.

Many traditional Western doctors still consider careful nutrition an 'alternative' rather than an essential approach to health — not surprising, considering the scant attention given to the subject in medical studies in the past.

To the Chinese teacher of physical fitness, whether in the martial arts, athletics and sport, or public health and healing, food is one of the first things considered along with improved breathing and exercise. A fairly typical commonsense list given by the Chin Wu school for the practice of Chi Kung is very similar, if not identical, to that given us by our local nutritionist – see the tables on page 213.

The Oriental believes the balance of physical and mental wholeness rests on these simple connections: when blood and energy are in harmony the nutrition and defensive energies are as one; the spirits will reside in the heart so that the quietness of the soul and the power of physical strength will be united; thus the human body is whole.

This may sound a little flowery but the philosophy was arrived at by some of the greatest students of the human state and its natural

THE FIVE FLAVOURS OF LIFE

FLAVOUR	ORGANS	EMOTION
Bitter	Heart	Joy to sorrow
Sour	Liver	Depression to anger
Sweet	Spleen	Sympathy to tolerance
Pungent	Lungs	Grief to despair
Salty	Kidneys	Timidity to fear

THE NATURAL FOODSTUFFS

GRAINS	FLAVOUR	ORGAN
Rice	Sweet	Good for spleen
Soya beans	Salty	Good for kidneys
Wheat*	Sour	Good for liver
Barley	Bitter	Good for heart
Millet	Pungent	Good for lungs

FRUITS		
Dates	Sweet	Good for spleen
Plums	Sour	Good for liver
Chestnuts	Salty	Good for kidneys
Almonds	Bitter	Good for heart
Peaches	Pungent	Good for lungs

VEGETABLES		
Marrow	Sweet	Good for spleen
Tomato	Sweet	Good for digestion
Sweet potato	Neutral–sweet	Good for kidneys
Lotus root**	Bitter	Good for heart
Onion	Pungent	Good for lungs

* Wheat grain, not wheat germ.

** Promotes 'lightheartedness'. It can be bought tinned or dried in any Chinese grocers.

ways who devoted lifetimes to its study and handed down their findings for others to take further. More often than not they were poor men, unable to afford court physicians and forced to discover cures and benefits in the fields and forests. These simple doctrines were devised in an age when life, though harsh, was less complicated and human beings were closer to the elements of nature. And is it really so obscure? How often do Westerners refer to a grumpy and irritable person as 'liverish' and to a joyful one as 'lighthearted'?

The Chinese also believed that the human state should be maintained in harmony with the seasons; because of the changes in temperature and climate one organ needs more nourishment than another at different times.

THE FOUR SEASONS

The seasons have always played a vital part in the Chinese calendar, both in the legendary festivals of the Twelve Moons and in down-to-earth attitudes to farming, fishing and medicine. Our lives, after all, are governed by climatic conditions. The constitution and physical needs of the Eskimo are entirely different from those of the African because they live in entirely different environments and respond to entirely different diets. The following relationships may once again seem little more than commonsense, but many of us would not recognise or follow them unless reminded.

The season relating to the liver is spring. The largest detoxification organ in the body, the liver needs to be prepared for the drastic change from the low temperature and warming foods of winter to the high temperature and cooling foods of summer. Sour flavours act as conditioners so that the extreme change will not prove too drastic. Spring is also the loosening-up stage for the tendons, ligaments and sinews, after the restrictions of winter and before the increased activity of summer.

The season relating to the heart is summer. Summer is the time of year when temperatures rise and the body needs cooling rather than overheating. Fresh foods, fruits, vegetables and salads are the order of the day, particularly for those whose circulation may be sluggish and who are therefore susceptible to heart problems.

The season relating to the lungs is autumn. The same principle applies to the transitional season of autumn as applies to spring. As temperatures begin to drop, the lungs need to prepare themselves for climatic change. Pungent or spicy foods act as conditioners.

The season relating to the kidneys is winter. In the winter the kidneys can easily become cold and damp — chilled — therefore cooling foods such as fresh fruit and vegetables are best avoided while soups, stocks and broths or other inner warming foods are beneficial, particularly for those who are heavy negative types.

A Chinese doctor will assess the condition of the vital organs by careful examination of the human face. After making a diagnosis the doctor will confirm his/her suspicions by checking the five pulses in the patient's wrist (yes, there are five pulses, not one; one for each of the five organs, or meridians (see pages 66–72)) which will tell the doctor the patient's internal condition in a matter of seconds. The next step is to prescribe corrective herbal medicine and adjust the diet. This skill was sorely tried in the Imperial courts of ancient China. When called to the bedside of an ailing female member of the royal family the doctor was not allowed to touch her, but was expected to read the five pulses through a ribbon tied to her wrist and emerging from under her bedcovers. If his diagnosis and treatment were not encouraging, neither were his chances for the future.

The Chinese attitude towards the five flavours brought into a modern context in terms of what to eat and what not to eat is summed up in the following list by Mr Chee Soo, President of the Chinese Cultural Arts Association in London. At first glance it may seem very restricting but there is little that contradicts the best Western dietary advice.

NOT ALLOWED:
♦ White bread, or anything made from white flour
♦ Refined or processed foods. If any colouring, preservatives, flavouring, chemicals or fruit acids are included, don't touch it.
♦ Fried food of any kind — grill it
♦ Coffee, alcohol, tobacco, chocolate
♦ Spices, rock salt, mustard, pepper, vinegar, pickles or curry
♦ Meat, red fish or blue fish
♦ White sugar
♦ Ice cream
♦ Potatoes or aubergines
♦ Concentrated meat extracts
♦ High fat cheese, whole milk or butter
♦ Birds or fish that have a lot of fat
♦ Lard or dripping

YOU MAY EAT THE FOLLOWING:
♦ Whole wheat or wholemeal bread, or anything made from wheat germ flour, soya flour, whole wheat or wholemeal flour
♦ Biscuits made from rye, barley, oats, wheat or corn flour
♦ Shredded wheat, muesli or similar breakfast foods, creamed rice, creamed oats, barley and rye
♦ Fresh vegetables and salads (raw and sautéed are best)
♦ Fresh fruit and berries
♦ Nuts (but not salted)
♦ Non-fat white fish, birds and poultry and seafoods
♦ Yoghurt (low fat)
♦ Powdered skim milk or skimmed milk
♦ Brown sugar or, better still, honey
♦ Cottage cheese or vegetarian cheese
♦ Weak tea or, better still, herb tea

♦ Vegetable margarine or oils, sesame oil or sunflower oil
♦ Fresh fruit drinks
♦ All dried fruit, apricots, prunes, raisins and currants
♦ Eggs, preferably scrambled or in omelettes

There are not many items in this commonsense list that do not coincide with Western standards apart from a few exceptions such as the reference to potatoes, a food seldom seen in China and replaced by rice in the everyday diet. Another aspect to be considered if you are to begin the practice of breathing exercises is that the internal nature of Chi Kung and its effect upon the major organs makes reconsideration of your eating habits an essential part of your new health program.

THE CHOLESTEROL STORY

The identification of cholesterol as a cardiovascular hazard has been established for over twenty years, but during that time, researchers have constantly changed their minds about the health problems associated with it. Among many other things, fatty fish such as sardines and mackerel, olive oil and avocados were once thought to raise blood cholesterol levels.

Now, scientists say these same foods can help lower and control those levels. The reason for the seemingly complete turnaround is the discovery that cholesterol takes several different forms. One of these is not only beneficial but essential for good health.

The body needs cholesterol to build cell membranes, produce certain hormones and promote metabolism and normal growth. Cholesterol is also one of the main elements of a substance called 'atheroma', which can cause narrowing of the arteries and reduce or cut off the blood supply to the organ or tissue beyond that narrowing. This is known as 'atherosclerosis'.

WHAT IS CHOLESTEROL?

A waxy, fat-like, tasteless, odourless substance, cholesterol is found mainly in fatty meats, eggs and butter, cream, offal and saturated animal fats in any form. Cholesterol is also manufactured in the human liver. It does not dissolve in blood plasma and our cells continually process it, wrapping it in water-soluble proteins which enable it to travel in the bloodstream.

Cholesterol is no longer regarded as a single, simple substance injurious to health. Two forms in particular are of primary importance to efficient bodily functions: LDL (low density lipoproteins) are considered harmful, for they can build up and clog arteries. HDL (high density lipoproteins) help move cholesterol through the system back to the liver, which begins digesting it. HDL are thought of as beneficial, for they help rid the body of excess LDL, cleaning out the fat that would otherwise build up on artery walls.

Researchers now agree that the body's balance of 'good' and 'bad' cholesterol — the HDL/LDL ratio, rather than the total cholesterol blood count — is the key to assessing a person's risk of cardiovascular disease. Therefore, the higher the HDL fraction, the higher the level of relative protection against the development of cardiovascular disease.

HEART PROBLEMS

It is now known that it is a combination of genes, attitude and diet that threatens the heart. Since we cannot do much about our genes, the only effective way of lowering our LDL levels is by adjusting our diet and outlook on life. Mainly, we should avoid saturated fat in all its well-disguised forms by not consuming more than 30 per cent of our total kilojoules in such foods as whole milk products, organ meats, heart, liver and kidney, poultry skin, squid, most shellfish, palm and coconut oils, brains, marbled beef, tripe, fat pork, bacon and sausages. Secondly, relieve stress. Present yourself with as much positive thought as reality will allow. Fight against negative influences and take time to relax. Some people need to 'retreat' and recharge to get a proper perspective of things. Others need to get out and about — to be doing things. No matter how you achieve it, a more relaxed and contented frame of mind — the ability to ride with the punches — will go a long way to help protect you from heart trouble.

A popular misconception is to eat less red meat but are replace it with a favourite substitute such as cheese. Hard cheeses or soft cheeses are just as fatty as each other. Cottage cheese on the other hand is not, but neither is it so tasty. Another misconception is about poultry meat; in fact, two pieces of fried chicken is 59 per cent saturated fat, against a Big Mac, which is 53 per cent fat.

EFFECTIVE BLOOD CLEANSERS

To support the blood-cleansing effects of oxygen circulation through breathing exercises, there are other excellent cleansers:

NIACIN Inhibits synthesis of a precursor of LDL in the liver and blocks triglyceride breakdown in fat tissues, reducing LDL and raising HDL. POSSIBLE SIDE EFFECTS Flushing, which could be very uncomfortable, perhaps dizziness, and itching. Some people report blurred vision. If any of these adverse effects is experienced, it may be best to reduce or stop the dosage.

ASPIRIN The usual aspirin tablet contains 325 milligrams. One tablet every other day is enough to help reduce the risk of fatty build-up. More will not increase the benefits but will probably increase the side effects. High doses can diminish the anti-clogging effects. Aspirin is best taken with food.

SIDE EFFECTS This common answer to headache or pain can cause internal bleeding and nausea. It is not recommended for people with ulcers and is not a magic cure-all. An aspirin every other day will not eliminate your cholesterol risk, but it can help if you exercise regularly and cut down on cigarettes and alcohol. A new low dose aspirin (Cardipin) has been developed (equivalent to approximately half a Disprin a day).

OMEGA 3 EPA (essential fatty acid found in fish oils) can help mobilise cholesterol by changing the composition of fatty acids. It can help bring down triglycerides (fat from land animals), by preventing platelets sticking together. Fish consumption (salmon and mackerel in particular) can reduce coronary heart disease by a factor of 2.5. It also has a anti-inflammatory effect, reducing morning stiffness and angina attack. Taken together with vitamin E, it increases the 'good' HDL cholesterol as vitamin E normalises deformability of red cells and is an important free radical scavenger. Together with vitamin C it is an effective anti-oxidant.

People on Aspirin or anti-coagulant therapy should check with their doctors before self-medicating with supplements of fish oil.

A very pleasant and extremely nourishing and more natural way of absorbing fish oil is through clear fish soup. If you do not find mackerel an easy fish to eat — it certainly isn't among the top tastes in fish — this recipe is easy to prepare, delicious to eat and very good for lowering or controlling cholesterol levels: Clean and wash two medium-sized mackerel (the slimy mackerel variety is best). Cut them in four and put the pieces (bones, heads and all) into a fair-sized soup pot. Add a good bunch of fresh watercress, a pinch of mixed herbs and a bay leaf. Bring to the boil and simmer for two hours. Drink the clear liquid hot. This is a very popular Chinese way of clearing the arteries and Ch'i channels.

SHOULD I HAVE A CHOLESTEROL TEST? It is suggested that adults over thirty years should have their serum cholesterol checked at least once every three to five years. If you think you belong to the possible high risk group, a screening would certainly be sensible. High risk factors are:
♦ A family history of coronary heart disease (especially if it has happened before turning fifty).
♦ Obesity.
♦ Smokers who don't exercise.
♦ Hypertension.
♦ Diabetes mellitus.
♦ Fatty deposits around the eyelids (if you are under forty).
♦ High fat and high salt diet (too much takeaway foods).

TWELVE WAYS TO PREVENT A HEART ATTACK

1 Watch your diet. Increased coronary mortality has been linked more and more with obesity. High blood pressure is more common in overweight people.

2 Include in your diet such green vegetables as brussels sprouts, cauliflower, broccoli, dried foods such as beans and peas, lentils, and oat bran. (Make sure vegetables are steamed or parboiled, raw as often as possible.)

3 Include fish in your diet, some excellent ones are tuna, mackerel, sardines and salmon, all have Omega 3 which helps to lower cholesterol and prevent blood clotting.

4 Cut down on fats and oils. Forty-two per cent of our calories come from fat. Decrease your intake of meat, butter, peanut butter, cream, egg yolks, organ meats, squid and shellfish.

5 Read the labels on tinned foods and, as much as possible, avoid processed foods and preserves. (That's not to say the occasional TV dinner or frozen snack will set you back but such convenience foods should be the exception rather than the rule.)

6 Niacin (a B group vitamin) is said to be helpful in inhibiting the liver's production of excessive cholesterol. Check with your doctor as you may develop a rash, other skin irritation or flushing.

7 Include garlic in your diet. Garlic, onions and raw carrots help reduce several forms of circulating cholesterol in the body.

8 Don't take yourself too seriously. Laughter involves biochemical endocrine and circulatory systems which in mysterious ways help to protect against heart problems.

9 Don't bottle up your feelings. Emotions such as anxiety, frustration, fury and rage have been linked to anginal pain. Working-out is one way of getting rid of many frustrations. Realise there is a way out and that you can change many aspects of your life.

10 Check your blood pressure regularly.

11 Include vitamin E and lecithin in your diet.

12 Try to cut down on smoking if you can't stop. Cigarette smoking appears to boost the bad LDL. The most positive way to increase the good HDL is aerobic activity for twenty to thirty minutes, at least three times a week.

Remember: Learn to breathe. Practise basic meditation as a form of 'cutting off' for stress relief and as a basis for relaxation. Restrict fat intake. Cut down on smoking. Moderate drinking. Enough exercise. Slow down ... avoid aggravation. Learn to distinguish the vital from the trivial in your everyday dealings. You might not live to 100, but life certainly will be more enjoyable!

DIET AND HEALTH

Obesity is a major public health problem in much of the industrialised world. Overweight people are at an increased risk of high blood pressure, arthritis, heart disease and diabetes. Crash diets not only upset the weight-control system but any sequence of severe kilojoule restriction can result in serious consequences which were not recognised until recently. Crash dieting, with its wide weight swings, is making people fat and unhealthy rather than slimmer and fitter.

The feast–fast cycle can cause a distinct form of high blood pressure. A 'dieter's hypertension' develops over a period of lose–gain fluctuations. This pattern could lead to congestive heart failure rather than the coronary heart attack or kidney disease common to other forms of hypertension.

In 1938, British scientists found that if laboratory rats were deprived of food and then allowed to eat normally, they became heavier than the rats that had never dieted. They called this rebound 'overcompensation'. When fat comes off too fast, protein tissue, firm muscle, organ and bone tissue are also lost, but when you regain weight it is largely fat. Cattle raisers capitalise on these findings by underfeeding their animals before fattening them.

Heredity protects some people from overcompensation, but the majority of dieters are not so fortunate. Overcompensation is kicked off by a deep dietary shock to the system. Fat cells shrink, although they never disappear. When normal eating starts the fat cells don't just fill up, they multiply and refill. For animals in the wild, threatened with periodic famine, such a biological system is their protection, but not for the ever-struggling dieter. The body can store more fat, and the next diet attempt will be more difficult.

HOW YOUR BODY CAN SABOTAGE YOUR EFFORTS

When your diet is nutritionally unsound and you are not obtaining enough kilojoules, your body not only loses valuable tissue, but you could suffer from the following:

SLEEP DISTURBANCE Carbohydrates are necessary to keep the brain's neurotransmitter, serotonin (needed for calmness and relaxation), high. When you deprive yourself, you feel edgy, anxious and irritable.

BAD BREATH Build-up of acids in the bloodstream (ketosis) and unneutralised hydrochloric acid are frequent causes.

FATIGUE Your body tries to conserve as much energy as possible by slowing down the production of hormones and enzymes that process it. Your store of sugars in the liver becomes depleted and your muscles lose size and of course, strength.

INDIGESTION When the normal food supply that neutralises stomach acids is cut drastically and suddenly, you can suffer indigestion from eating too little.

HYPERTENSION The yoyo syndrome of crash dieting causes an increase in the body's stress hormone, norepinephrine, which constricts blood vessels and can increase blood pressure. If weight remains constant, blood pressure raised in this way will return to normal in two years.

How to Beat the Weight Boomerang

The critical factor in breaking out of this cycle is not another crash diet. Dieter's hypertension will disappear with time if you keep your weight constant, either higher or lower. Recovery takes about two years.

A kilogram of fat is equivalent to about 29 000 kilojoules. So, in order to shed one kilogram of fat, you will have to burn 29 000 kilojoules more than is required to maintain your current weight. A daily deficit of, say, 2000 kilojoules should enable you to lose half a kilogram per week. The answer, then, is exercise.

Physical activity slowly and subtly resets the systems that control metabolism and regulate weight. Exercise can actually lower the dieter's high blood pressure in part by slowing norepinephrine production. Norepinephrine is your 'fight or flight' hormone, which speeds up heart beat and raises blood pressure. When you over-indulge, your norepinephrine output will increase. Overfeeding, in anyone, can lead to increases in blood pressure.

Exercise can also strengthen the heart, which may have been weakened by protein loss during too many years of experimental dieting. Although increasing physical activity is a great help in shedding excess kilograms, reduced food intake is the main factor in a successful weight-loss program.

Long-term modification of both your food intake and energy expenditure are necessary for maintaining normal body-weight. For most individuals in less-than-active jobs, it is rather a case of too little physical activity than too much food. However, if you are serious about losing weight, make modest cuts in your daily intake (say up to 1000 kilojoules a day), which isn't too much of a sacrifice.

Include any of the activities mentioned under exercise — brisk walking, dancing, swimming, cycling or jogging for thirty minutes every other day and you can achieve 'residual metabolic elevation', burning off an extra 200 to 400 kilojoules in the four hours after exercise. Some experts say that exercising between 4 p.m. and 8 p.m. is therefore the most effective.

ARE THERE MIRACLE FOODS?

Nutrition is a comparatively new science and susceptible to fads and cults. 'Health' foods are supposed to be beneficial. 'Natural' foods supposedly comprise of products made and marketed with a minimum of processing without use of any artificial ingredients or preservatives, and are often promoted as having health-giving and curative properties.

There are no miracle foods. Yeast and wheat germ, for example, are nutritious but cannot cure ailments on their own. There is so much confusing information that it is little wonder most of us do not know what to believe.

The important thing is to take care in your shopping. Many packaged 'health' foods contain additives (flavouring, colouring, sulphur dioxide, sorbic acid and so on — as in all dried tree fruit). It is important to read the labels carefully. Some, of course, are inadequately labelled, in which case, if in doubt, try another brand that is more open about its ingredients.

No single food can make you slim. And no special foods alone have curative powers or alone provide the energy to improve physical performance or psychological stability. Bearing this in mind, the suggested foods that follow are rich in vitamins and minerals and can help to promote better health and increase vitality. But they are not cure-alls. Better nutrition cannot cure ailments, but poor eating habits will adversely affect every condition no matter how severe or slight.

WHEAT GERM — AN OLD FAVOURITE The heart of the wheat kernel, wheat germ is rich in vitamin E, and minerals such as magnesium, calcium, manganese, phosphorus and copper. Sprinkle on yoghurt or muesli. It needs refrigeration in a tightly closed container as the oil in it oxidises and can go rancid. A tablespoon per day is ample as it is rich in fat.

GARLIC — NOT JUST AN OLD WIVES' TALE Some people object to the smell of garlic, but it is a powerful detoxicant, and can help to clear fat accumulation from the blood vessels, lower cholesterol and protect against bacterial and viral infections. (Don't use raw garlic as it can burn the tissues of the stomach and small intestine walls, causing inflammation, resulting in burping or repeating). Garlic has been used throughout history to help combat the degenerative processes of ageing because of its unique properties:

- It helps lower serum cholesterol and can help prevent arterio-sclerosis.
- It clears waste from the system and renders some toxic substances harmless.
- It helps to maintain body resistance to mild infections and is valuable for the temporary relief of mucus and congestion during colds, bronchitis, sinusitis or catarrh, and other respiratory conditions.
- It can also be used as an antiseptic tonic, for it has antibiotic, antifungal and antibacterial qualities.
- Garlic also has a beneficial influence on the arteries and heart functions.

Garlic does give off a distinctive, pungent odour when crushed, due to the disulphides and allicin. It is one of the most widely used kitchen herbs and its distinctive characteristics are the primary reasons for its popularity.

Its stimulating effect on the digestive system and consequent ability to improve poor digestion has made it popular for some 3000 years. Nowadays, many people believe it is useful to prevent stomach upsets while travelling, when changes of diet, climate and water can be disturbing. Garlic is a good source of many minerals (including selenium and sulphur) and amino acids; capsules or tablets are convenient for use as a daily supplement. People with degenerative conditions of the liver, gall-bladder, bile duct or pancreas should not use garlic medicinally as garlic stimulates the bile flow and can make a person feel nauseated. Also, too much raw garlic can also cause anaemia by oxidising the red blood cells.

LIVE SPROUTS — FRESH AND EASY Sprouts can be grown on your windowsill, in the laundry, or any cool shaded part of the house. They provide minerals, complex carbohydrates, vitamins and some essential fatty acids. Add sprouts to salads or yoghurt or use as toast and sandwich toppings. They are low in calories and generally pleasant tasting. Sprouts most readily available are alfalfa, wholewheat, mung beans, millet, rye and fenugreek, to mention only a few.

KELP — A WONDER FROM THE SEA Kelp, an edible seaweed, is a good source of iodine, can help strengthen nails and hair and is rich in B-complex vitamins and vitamins D, E and K, as well as calcium and magnesium. It is an excellent addition to soups, salads or casseroles.

SEEDS — ANOTHER INTERNATIONAL FAVOURITE Sesame, sunflower and pumpkin seeds are excellent sources of protein. Ground in a blender, a mixture can be sprinkled on salads, sandwiches, fruit and yoghurt, or nibbled anytime, anywhere.

Sesame seeds are rich in calcium, magnesium and potassium. They contain more calcium than cheese, milk or nuts. Sunflower seeds are rich in vitamin E and iron and B-complex vitamins as well as zinc and magnesium, which makes them particularly helpful for stress relief.

Pumpkin seeds are high in B vitamins, iron and zinc and are said to have strong antiparasitic properties.

YOGHURT — THE ANSWER TO DAIRY PRODUCTS A plain non-fat yoghurt will supply your body with calcium, riboflavin and protein. It also benefits the digestive system by keeping the intestines clean. The bacteria in yoghurt are antagonistic to putrefying bacteria that can cause toxicity in your body. Yoghurt contains a mixture of lacto-bacillus acidophilus and other bacteria and is a good source of B vitamins. Yoghurt can also help restore the balance of natural intestinal flora disturbed by antibiotics.

Commercially made fruit yoghurt, however, contains too much sugar and fat.

FAD DIETS — SUCCESS AND FAILURE

Any diet that suddenly becomes temporarily popular is generally considered a fad. Over the years, there have been many fad diets, ranging from the ice cream diet, the nut diet, the grape diet, the vegetable diet, to the 'Hollywood' diet of little more than a hard-boiled egg and half a grapefruit. Some permit you to eat all you want of one or two foods. Theoretically, you will get thoroughly fed-up with the limited choice and the monotony will make you eat less and eventually lose weight.

Diets like these are nutritionally unbalanced and too monotonous for any but the fanatic to tolerate. Even if you do lose weight, you won't have developed new eating habits; when you resume your former eating habits, you'll soon regain weight.

In a recent survey of 15 000 readers of a major women's magazine, 42 per cent of the overweight readers confessed to being on-again/off-again dieters. All agreed that pills, crash diets, hypnosis and acupuncture worked to some extent, but not for long. Weight control is a constant struggle that can only be resolved through a sensible approach to eating, cutting down on fat-foods and, above all, continuing regular exercise.

Crash dieting sets up a pattern of weight loss and rebound gain that can make the itinerate dieter even heavier. This is how it works: when you severely restrict your food intake, you force your body to adjust to the onset of starvation conditions. But nature is a wonderful thing — it takes care of itself. Your body conserves energy by lowering the metabolic rate. This sets the stage for renewed weight gain as soon as you eat normally. The starve–feast cycle can turn a moderately overweight person into a very overweight one.

THOUGHTS FOR A COMMONSENSE WEIGHT-LOSS PROGRAM

If dieting were easy, no one would be overweight, but dieting is thwarted at every turn by nature's determination to protect us from starvation. Many strict diets can make us cranky, hungry and nervous. Here are two workable approaches that might suit your lifestyle.

Each kilogram of body fat amounts to 29 000 kilojoules of stored energy. Dieting forces us to use stored fat to meet our energy needs when the food we eat is reduced. Everyone burns up kilojoules just keeping the body functioning, even when asleep.

Most adult women need an average of about 8000 kilojoules a day. In order to burn stored fat, the only way is to decrease your daily food intake. An active man can burn off (metabolise) more kilojoules than a woman and does not need to watch his intake so carefully.

CUT DOWN IN ALL DIRECTIONS

In this plan, you do not have to eliminate anything. You don't have to weigh, measure and plan your meals like a military operation. You lose weight simply by eating less. Together with this rather obvious procedure, you double your activity whilst halving your daily food intake.

Most nutritionists agree that this is the healthiest way. It is not a severely limiting program and is neither monotonous nor impracticable. However, your meals must be nutritionally balanced and not overloaded with snacks and fatty foods. As we need 8000 kilojoules a day to maintain our weight, the only way to lose those centimetres is to cut down to 4000 kilojoules a day — and exercise.

Try to include foods from each of the five main groups: Protein, fruit and vegetables, dairy products, grains (cereals and bread), but limiting butter and oils. (See the top twenty hit list of fattening foods, pages 233.)

If you intend to take on a strenuous exercise program whilst cutting down on your food intake, you may be wiser to allow an additional 1000 to 1200 kilojoules per day in order to maintain good health.

At this rate, the weight loss will not be sudden and spasmodic. It will be a steady loss of say a half to one kilogram per week or a little more if you exercise vigorously. (See exercise chart, page 180).

If you can stay with this diet, you are bound to lose weight. And because you do get to eat a little of everything, you won't feel deprived, short-changed or bored. Therefore, you are less likely to break out and go on a binge. It is a diet you can actually stay with, by simply exercising moderate discipline.

Don't expect to see results on a daily basis. It is not a good idea to weigh yourself more than once a week, for although you may lose several kilograms initially, later weight loss will probably be steady rather than drastic.

THE DIET DIARY

This is more a weight-loss tool rather than an actual diet plan. 'Behaviour restructuring' concentrates on why and how you eat rather than on what you eat. It depends on the fact that we all have certain eating patterns established over many years, which need rearranging if we are overweight. It requires honesty on your part and discipline in confronting your bad eating habits by keeping a food diary recording everything you put in your mouth.

You have to write down everything you eat to understand your special cravings and needs. When you see everything in black and white without the usual vagueness often associated with cheating, you then realise how much you are eating and this can act as a motivating factor — 'Wow, do I really eat that much?'

List what you eat as well as when, where, with whom and why, that is, were you bored, upset, frustrated, nervous, tired, cold or hungry? Or were you keeping someone else company although you may not have planned to eat at that time? Could you have done just as well without it?

A word of warning. Keeping a food diary can be tedious and laborious, but it has also proved very effective. It brings you into direct confrontation with your enemy. If you feel embarrassed about your eating habits, don't leave your diary where others can see it. After all, it's your problem and your business. This way, you won't be tempted to leave anything out. If this plan sounds dubious to you, remind yourself that most schools of modern psychology advise the writing down of problems as the best form of confrontation and resolve.

It may take a few weeks before you can see a pattern emerging from your private assessment. The most obvious goal is to learn to eat only when you feel hungry. If your diary shows that your main problem is nibbling snacks when you have nothing to do, reduce the temptation by doing something with your hands, for example, any simple housework, or going for a walk. Develop a craft or hobby as a standby for such circumstances or, if you're feeling energetic enough, some heavy work in the garden will keep you away from the kilojoules.

Eating slowly helps. It takes some twenty minutes for your body to signal your brain that you've eaten enough. By the time you've waited twenty minutes, you may not want that second helping.

It is not a good idea to gulp down anything while standing up and doing something else at the same time. Eating while you're active can make you eat more than you realise. One of the most important things we can learn from Asia is the very civilised ritual of enjoying food — an age-old outlook that sees eating as the ultimate relaxation, not to be hurried or disturbed by anything but the company and conversation of family or friends.

Accept that keeping a food diary will probably be boring. Don't be too hard on yourself; introducing new eating restrictions, no matter how limited, isn't that simple and takes a little time to get used to. Don't expect to see results immediately or to lose weight drastically. Fast weight-loss fad diets are at best temporary and often nutritionally unbalanced, but behaviour modification can have long-lasting and pleasing results. Once you get used to it as part of your routine it will not be difficult to maintain.

DON'T DEPRIVE YOURSELF OF CARBO-HYDRATES

It seems that most weight-loss programs restrict the intake of carbohydrates, because eating sugars and starches blocks the fat-burning process. At the same time, low carbohydrate intake can eventually lower your level of serotonin, the chemical messenger in the brain that is a relaxant and appetite regulator. When the serotonin level is low you feel hungry, and the only effective way to get the level back up again is to increase carbohydrates.

Most people are not satisfied with their current weight, whether it is those stubborn few kilograms or a more serious excess, so by cutting down on bread, cereals, potatoes and the like, many are in fact walking around in a mild to severe state of carbohydrate deprivation. Our brain serotonin levels become low and our carbohydrate receptors clamour for nourishment. The more strict your diet, the more you are likely to go on a binge and head for the nearest pastry shop.

A possible biochemical explanation of our appetite for iced Danish, toasted bread with honey, cakes, croissants and sweets generally is that carbohydrates have a tranquillising effect. Nobody secretly pigs out on carrot or celery sticks. Carbohydrates raise your blood sugar almost immediately, flooding the system with instant insulin; and then you feel sluggish again. The cause is a rise in serotonin, that home-grown tranquilliser and appetite regulator.

The amino acid tryptophan is used by the brain, with the help of vitamin B6, to produce serotonin, which has a sedative effect, hence tryptophan's recommendation for promoting sleep.

Tryptophan is an essential amino acid. Your body cannot manufacture it. You can buy it without prescription from chemists or health stores. It seems that tryptophan may alleviate stress, anxiety and depression and could be an aid for the dieter, helping you avoid the false soothing and nurturing aspects of secret binging, followed afterwards by the inevitable guilt and anger.

But take heart even if you do decide to kick stress in the teeth occasionally by indulging in your favourite forbidden foods. We restrain our real selves so often in so many areas of our lives, breaking the rules sometimes actually fulfils many complex needs — biochemical and emotional.

DIETING DOS AND DON'TS

♦ *Do* eat regularly. If you don't eat, you'll be slimmer but not healthier. So *don't* skip meals. When you go too long without food, you'll eventually give up and probably eat too much as compensation. So, see that you eat regular and balanced meals.

♦ *Do* be discriminating about your treats. If the pastry or cake you bite into is really not the best or freshest you can get, you have the option of throwing it in the rubbish bin. Don't waste your precious kilojoules on less than the best.

♦ *Do* keep occupied. If you are bored, turn to alternative activities. Wash your hair, go shopping, ring a friend, write a letter, start a project inside or out, instead of heading for the kitchen and certain temptation.

♦ *Do* drink more water. A large glass of water before a party is an effective habit to get into. It may not be satisfying but it helps take the edge off your appetite.

♦ *Do* use only non-stick cookware. Every 30 grams of butter and margarine amounts to 920 kilojoules; 30 millilitres of oil costs you 1110 kilojoules. Non-stick helps you to use the bare minimum.

♦ *Do* avoid sugar whenever possible. Sugar has no vitamins or valuable minerals. Empty kilojoules are nice enough to the taste, but do not good at all for the body.

- *Do* eat fruit rather than drink juice. This may not be so convenient but it gives essential fibre that is otherwise wasted.
- *Do* rediscover salads. There are some wonderful combinations to add to you meals. It is a low kilojoule filler high in nutrition, but hold the condiments, mayonnaise and oil.
- *Do* say no to second helpings. Resist the temptation to have a little more. If you can't say no to more than you need you're unlikely to survive any diet plan.
- *Do* get used to clear soups rather than cream soups. One bowl of cream soup has more kilojoules than several bowls of clear.
- *Do* brush your teeth often. The fresh taste can help take away your desire to nibble again.
- *Do* shop for groceries as infrequently as possible. Supermarket shelves present temptations that can be hard to resist, especially on an 'off day'. Wander into clothes shops and department stores in your lunch hour and stay away from the tantalising aromas of fast food.
- *Do* reward yourself. If you've made a little progress, go out and buy something nice (other than food) for yourself. You deserve it. Give away your 'fat' clothes — sacks, tents or clothes with elastic waist-bands — they allow you to put on centimetres and still feel comfortable. Buy something flattering.
- *Do* burn up kilojoules whenever you can. Use the stairs instead of the lift. Get off the bus a couple of stops earlier, walk at lunchtime.

- *Don't* attempt to start dieting while trying to break another habit, or while under any emotional stress. For instance, don't try to give up smoking or drinking at the same time as dieting. It's asking too much of yourself and would be too much of a strain on even the strongest resources. When you have overcome one, you will be more confident and able to tackle the next. If you find yourself under severe emotional pressure, moving house, changing jobs, separation from a loved one, any kind of loss, it's not a good time to impose further demands on yourself.
- *Don't* tempt yourself by testing your willpower. If you had a lot of that elusive commodity in the first place, you wouldn't be dieting now. So keep junk food at arm's length or out of your house altogether. Get rid of risky foods and *don't* replace them.
- *Don't* weigh yourself alone, get disappointed and then worry. This has proved the end of many a good intention. Get involved in activities that keep your morale up. It is much easier to tackle a diet when you feel good about yourself.
- *Don't* be disappointed if others don't seem to notice your accomplishments. Some people may be quite hostile to successful

weight losers, but you are the only one who really knows what you have achieved and that's all that matters. It's your life, your body, your decision.

- *Don't* let the guilt of the occasional slip destroy your diet. One lapse doesn't mean defeat. If you must break routine, try to do it on the same day every week.
- *Don't* feel you have to make up excuses to hide the fact that you are dieting. You have a right to be healthy and fit, to look and feel your best; criticism is probably jealousy. Keep your diet to yourself. The less you talk about it, the more you are likely to stick to it.
- *Don't* go shopping on an empty stomach, especially when you are tired, or feeling run down. You are likely to buy more than you need, especially sweets, snacks and convenience meals.
- *Don't* go shopping without a list, and make sure it doesn't include things you know you shouldn't eat. The list will guide you past the possibility of impulse buying, so stick to it.
- *Don't* chew gum. It can actually make you hungry by stimulating the salivary glands. Gum chewing doesn't really help calm your nerves although you may think it does, so there are no real advantages.
- *Don't* skip breakfast. You'll be so hungry by mid-morning, you'll probably find yourself longing for a doughnut or a Danish. If you manage to get through to lunchtime, you'll be hungry enough to head for the nearest fast food you can find and probably end up overeating.
- *Don't* eat too quickly. It is the amount of food in the blood rather than in the stomach that triggers the stop signal when you've had enough to satisfy your body's needs. But it takes time for that food to digest and be absorbed into the bloodstream. If you eat too fast you can finish the equivalent of two meals before your brain tells you that you're no longer hungry. Another advantage of eating more slowly is that you can taste and enjoy what you eat.
- *Don't* eat standing up. Stand-up-eating is speed eating. It also makes you feel as though you haven't had a satisfying meal no matter how much you may have swallowed.
- *Don't* think of yourself as being on a diet. As soon as you admit you are depriving yourself, you'll be tempted to cheat. Tell yourself you are doing your one and only body a big favour and remind yourself of all the rewards.
- *Don't* serve up an entire meal at once. Served together, a three-course meal somehow looks less than it is. It's best to help yourself in the kitchen and carry your plate to the table leaving the rest out of sight. By leaving the serving dishes on the table you run a bigger risk of helping yourself to that second helping that you don't really need.

1 Dark chocolate 120 kJ (29 cal.) a square.
   Milk chocolate 570 kJ (135 cal.) per 25 g (about 6 squares).

2 Nuts (with the exception of chestnuts):
   Peanuts, 50 g small packet has 1215 kJ (289 cal.);.
   Cashews, 50 g has 1200 kJ (285 cal.);
   Macadamias, 50 g has 1480 kJ (352 cal.).

3 Potato crisps, a small 25 g packet will cost you 600 kJ (142 cal.).

4 Mayonnaise, 1 tablespoon can ruin your good salad intentions at 600 kJ (142 cal.).

5 Peanut butter has 750 kJ (179 cal.) to the tablespoon.

6 Butter and margarine have 610 kJ (145 cal.) to the tablespoon. If you use about a teaspoon, it'll cost you 150 kJ (36 cal.).

7 Oil has a massive 740 kJ (176 cal.) per tablespoon and 185 kJ (44 cal.) per teaspoon.

8 Lard is your worst enemy: 755 kJ (180 cal.) per tablespoon.

9 Bacon is 605 kJ (144 cal.) per 25 g (that's about half a rasher).

10 Shortbread, 25 g has 545 kJ (120 cal.).

11 Toffee, 470 kJ (112 cal.) in every 25 g.

12 Sausage rolls and meat pies, 395 kJ (94 cal.) per 25 g.

13 Cream cheese, 435 kJ (103 cal.) per 25 g.

14 Salami, 425 kJ (101 cal.) per 25 g (about 2 pieces).

15 Cheeses: Gruyère cheese, 490 kJ (117 cal.) for 25 g;
   Boursin, 485 kJ (115 cal.) for 25 g;
   Blue stilton, 545 kJ (130 cal.) for 25 g;
   Parmesan, 485 kJ (115 cal.) per 25 g or 105 kJ (25 cal.) per teaspoon.

16 Sesame bar (health food), 470 kJ (111 cal.) per 25 g.

17 Pastry, 420 kJ (100 cal.) for 25 g.

18 Fruit cake, 100 g slice has 1690 kJ (402 cal.) or 420 kJ (100 cal.) for 25 g.

19 Frankfurts, 756 kJ (180 cal.) per 30 g.

20 Pâté, 567 kJ (135 cal.) per 30 g.

Here are some questions that might give you food for thought — instead of the other kind. If you can answer all ten of them correctly, you are already well advanced in basic nutrition.

FOOD FACTS OR FADS

Q. When on a diet, should I drink fewer liquids?
A. No. Water, or any kind of liquid, is important for body function. If you cut down your liquid consumption, your weight loss will be water loss not fat loss and the risk of dehydration will be greater. On the other hand, if you drink more than you need, your body will soon get rid of it.

Q. Will drinking a glass of milk before drinking alcohol prevent me from getting drunk?

A. You can be affected by alcohol a lot more quickly on an empty stomach, as it is immediately absorbed into the bloodstream. Fatty food in the stomach stops alcohol from being absorbed as quickly. Although a glass of milk won't stop you getting drunk it can at least slow the process.

Q. Is toast less fattening than bread?

A. No. Toast weighs a little less than untoasted bread due to some moisture loss in the toasting process but both have the same kilojoule value. In fact, as butter or margarine often melts into toast, you are probably using more than you would on untoasted bread.

Q. Does smoking a cigarette after a meal help digestion?

A. Definitely not. Smoking does not help anything other than give you something to do with your hands when under pressure.

Q. Do carrots help you see better in the dark?

A. Carrots contain carotene which changes into vitamin A in your body. If you are low on vitamin A, eating carrots will improve your ability to see in dim light. If you are not deficient, extra carotene will do very little for your eyes.

Q. Are brown eggs better for me than white eggs?

A. The colour of the shell does not make any difference, but free-range eggs are probably better than battery eggs.

Q. Is brown bread better for me than white bread?

A. As a rule, yes. But be careful what brand you choose, some breads are 'tinted'. Wholemeal breads contain more vitamin B and iron and some have more protein. White bread contains about 8.5 per cent protein. We eat so much bread that it really is worth taking the time to read bread wrappers carefully.

Q. Is brown sugar better for me than white sugar?

A. The darkest brown sugar contains about 2.5 mg iron and 35 mg of calcium per 100 g whilst there is no calcium or iron in white sugar. But the quantity is so small, there is hardly any difference worth considering; sugar is sugar and while we all need a certain amount of it we should reduce our intake.

Q. Is margarine less fattening than butter?

A. They both contain equal kilojoules.

Q. Will yoghurt help me lose weight?

A. Yoghurt is very similar nutritionally to milk, from which it is made. The low-fat yoghurts are lower in kilojoules and fats. Fruit yoghurts are generally sweetened with sugar, even if only fruit sugar, and therefore can be a trap. Unsweetened — no fruit — low-fat yoghurts are certainly your best bet.

THE MIDRIFF CRISIS

Most of us will face the reality of the thickening waistline. The midriff crisis is probably going to be part and parcel of the midlife crisis, if you choose to see it in that light. Unless, of course, you tend towards the ectomorphic body type — in which case, nothing is going to make you stack it on where most of us do — or, unless you really are a dedicated exerciser who pays particular attention to the mid-section with prolonged and regular abdominal work — you'll probably lose the waist war.

But being big around the middle doesn't necessarily mean being weak and soft and it certainly doesn't mean being inflexible. In fact, you can be just as fit and well as someone much slimmer if you accept the wider waistline for what it is and work at reducing it. Whether you succeed or not, as long as the stomach muscles are toned up and doing their very important job of relieving the back from doing all the work, you will have won the main battle.

No matter what your measurements around the waist, the vital thing is firmness, tighter abdominal muscles, which means a more efficient gut, inside and out. The tendency is to give up in despair, but dieting combined with waist and abdominal exercise will definitely tighten things up and it may reduce the centimetres. But if you don't see diet as part of your personal answer, at least you will have to begin giving your waist some work. If you don't, it will just get bigger and softer, and there's nothing more demoralising if you care about how you look and how you feel.

Chinese Chi Kung practitioners may quite often posses very generous midriffs, brought about by continuous sinking of the Ch'i (and probably continuous enjoyment of rice and noodles), but they are hard as iron. Powerful enough to bounce an opponent six metres if summoned to do so. Many a fool has sprained a wrist by driving a blow into what looked like a large and flabby stomach.

Here are some abdominal exercises which if fitted into your breathing routine will make you feel much better about that part of you that tries so hard to get away.

ABDOMINAL EXERCISES

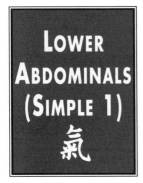

LOWER ABDOMINALS (SIMPLE 1)

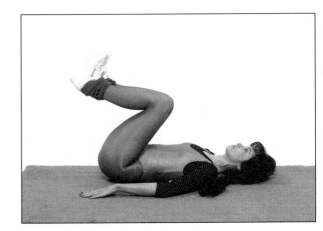

STEP 1 ▶

Lie on your back with your head on the floor. Bring both knees towards your chest. Keep your feet flexed and your knees together.

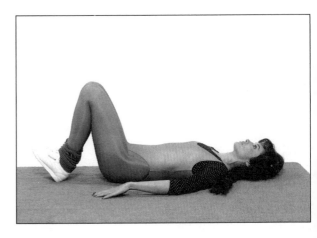

STEP 2 ▶

Bring your heels down as close as possible to your buttocks, keeping your knees together. Return your knees to the chest and repeat eight times.

CAUTION Keep your head on the floor. Do not tense your neck and shoulders. Do not arch your back. Do not hold your breath.

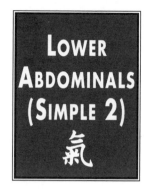
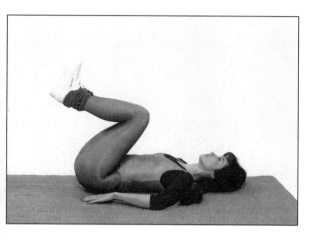

◄ **S T E P   1**

Lie on your back, lower back pressed against the floor. Bring both knees towards your chest. Keep your feet flexed.

S T E P   2 ►

Push your legs out (45°). Do not straighten completely. Keep your feet flexed as if pushing at the wall in front of you. Repeat eight times.

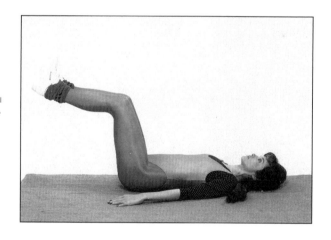

CAUTION Your head should remain on the floor. Do not arch your back. Do not hold your breath.

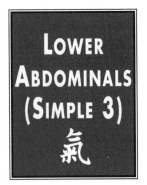

LOWER ABDOMINALS (SIMPLE 3)

CAUTION Support your neck but do not push your head forward. Knees must be bent to prevent any strain on the lower back. Elbows are out to the side, keeping the shoulder-blades off the floor. If you experience tension in the neck, make a cradle with your arms for support. Exhale when you lift up. Inhale when you relax.

STEP 1 ▶

Lie on your back with your feet flat on the floor. Support your neck with your hands. Look up at the ceiling and lift your head off the floor. Lower your head without actually touching the floor. Repeat eight times.

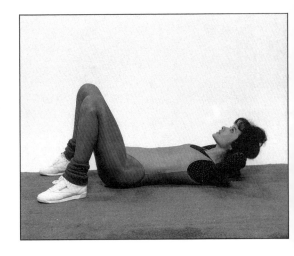

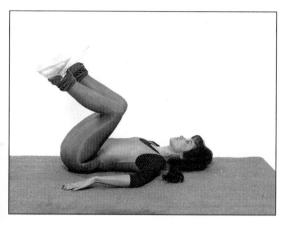

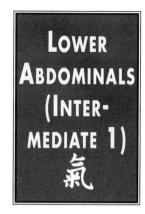

LOWER ABDOMINALS (INTERMEDIATE 1)
氣

STEP 1 ▲

Lie on your back with your head on the floor, legs apart. Bring both knees towards your chest. Keep your feet flexed.

STEP 2 ▶

Bring your heels down as close as possible to your buttocks. Return your knees to your chest. Repeat eight times.

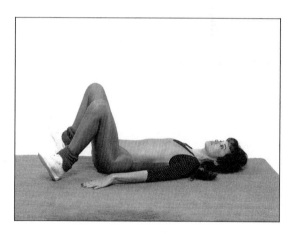

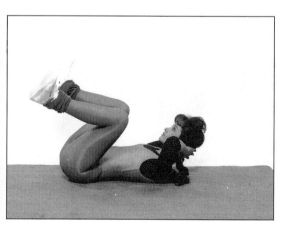

◀ STEP 3

To work the upper body at the same time, lift your torso as you lift your knees towards your chest. Support your neck with both hands. Do not lower your head to touch the floor. Repeat eight times.

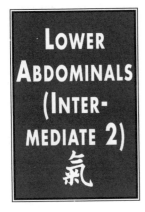
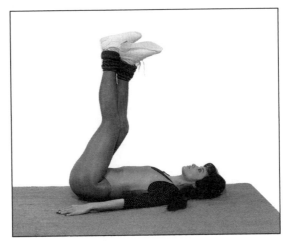

STEP 1 ▲

Lie on your back with your head on the floor. Lift your legs towards the ceiling and cross at the ankles. The feet are flexed.

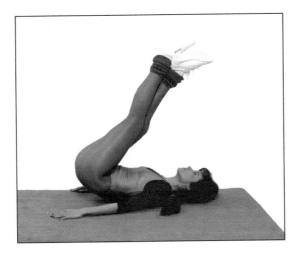

◄ **STEP 2**

Lift your bottom off the floor, pushing your feet towards the ceiling. Return to starting position and repeat eight times.

CAUTION Don't hold your breath. Keep your head on the floor. When you lift the legs, do not bring them back behind your head.

CAUTION: As with all abdominal exercises, do not hold your breath. Support your neck without forcing your head forward.

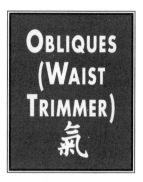

OBLIQUES (WAIST TRIMMER) 氣

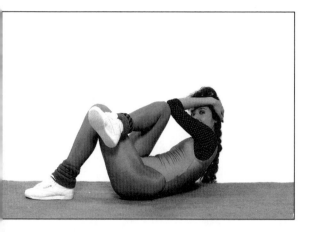

◀ S T E P 1

Lie on your back, bend your left knee, with the foot flat to the floor. Bring the right ankle across your bent left knee. Support your neck with your left hand. Extend your right arm on the floor. Lift up and bring your left elbow to your right knee. Repeat eight times. Try it on the opposite side.

CAUTION: Do not arch your back. Keep both knees bent to prevent lower back strain. Breathe rhythmically.

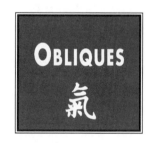

OBLIQUES 氣

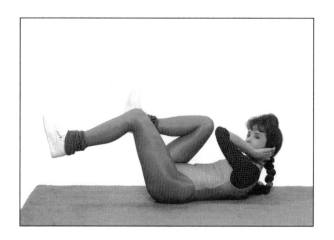

◀ S T E P 1

Lie on your back, supporting your neck with your hands. Lift and twist the body to allow your elbow to touch the opposite knee. Repeat on the opposite side. Do this exercise eight times on each side, preferably to music to make it easier. This works the rectus abdominis (long central muscle) as well as the obliques (running along the sides).

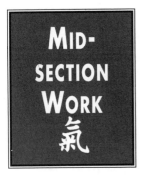

MID-SECTION WORK 氣

STEP 1 ▶

Lie on your back with one knee bent, and the foot flat on the floor. Extend the other leg towards the ceiling. Support the back of the neck if your abdominals are not very strong. Touch the opposite foot with extended hand. Repeat eight times. Try the same exercise on the opposite side.

CAUTION Avoid rounding the shoulders. Support the neck if it is uncomfortable, making sure the abdominals are doing the work. Make sure the knee is bent at all times to prevent strain on the lower back.

NOTE If this is easy, add half kilogram hand-weights as you reach for the opposite foot.

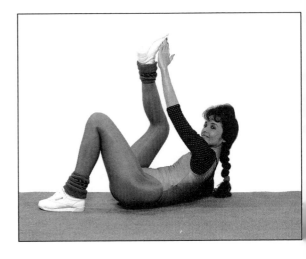

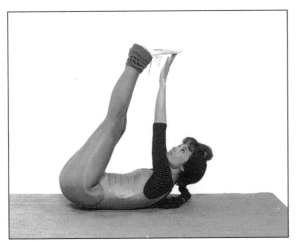

◀ STEP 2

Lie on the floor with your feet flexed and extended towards the ceiling. Reach both hands towards your toes as you lift your torso. Repeat eight times.

NOTE If this is too difficult, support your neck with one hand and stretch the other one towards the toes. Alternate the movement.

This is a good abdominal and thigh strengthener. It is an advanced exercise and should be done only if you have no lower back problems.

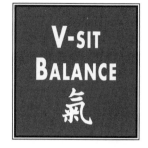

V-SIT
BALANCE
氣

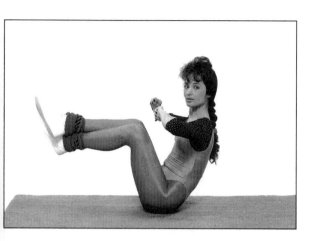

S T E P S   1 & 2   ▲ ▶

Balance on your buttocks. Lift your legs off the floor, with your knees slightly bent. Cross them at the ankles, with the calves parallel to the floor. Arms can be bent or extended. Or punch it out, working the shoulders as well. Hold for a slow count of four. Repeat the exercise six times.

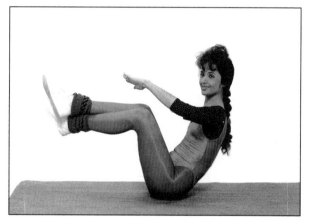

CAUTION Do not arch your back. Make sure there isn't anything behind you, in case you fall backwards.

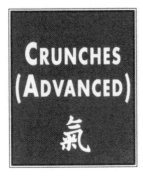

CRUNCHES (ADVANCED)

氣

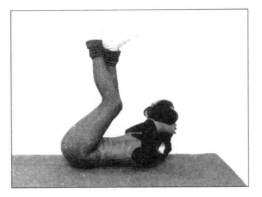

STEP 1 ▲

Lie on the floor with both legs extended towards the ceiling and your feet flexed. Cross at the knees, which are slightly bent so that the lower back does not arch. Support your neck with your hands. Lift up towards your knees and exhale. Keep your shoulder-blades off the floor. Inhale and lower your head, but do not lie back on the floor. This strengthens the thighs as well as the abdominals.

CAUTION The knees are slightly bent to prevent lower back strain.
NOTE Tighten the abdominal muscles as you lift.

MEDITATION AND CH'I

There are but three ways,
the way of the Heavens,
the way of the Earth,
and the way we must follow, the Tao

Lin Tui

PART
ELEVEN

MEDITATION AND CH'I

Most forms of physical discipline practised in Asia have a strong connection with meditation. The further one goes into the study of self-mastery, the more important control of the mind becomes. No great Master of the past reached the ultimate goal without bringing thoughts and emotions to heel. They believed that if the untrained body was as erratic in its movements as the untrained mind, we would be lucky to come through a day unscathed — not an exaggeration when we consider the tangents our minds so often take without rhyme or reason and think of the consequences if our bodies behaved in a similar way. Most of us would be lucky to get from one side of the road to the other, let alone survive behind the wheel of a car.

So, the great Masters believed a trained body was impossible without a trained mind. In this sense meditation was used to store and release energy at will, to conserve Ch'i and to unleash it with speed and power. This phenomenon is illustrated in its purest form by the almost superhuman feats demonstrated by the advanced external, or 'hard style', martial artist. The shattering of bricks and roof tiles, piercing of boards and buckling of metal with the foot or fist are not tricks. They are achieved by total concentration of mind, body and breath, concentrated upon the single spot and the single thought until nothing else exists in the universe except the strike. The often terrifying sound that accompanies such great effort is caused by the sudden release of breath rather than a will to impress onlookers. This harness of power is far too violent for our simple purpose of improved breathing.

Related to breath control and the development of Ch'i, meditation is also relevant to Pa Tuan Tsin. Any effective fitness routine calls for total concentration. It is utterly useless to approach a half hour of relaxing exercise with a racing mind that cannot be stilled.

Various kinds of meditation are nowadays prescribed as readily as enemas and emetics. Unfortunately, relief through meditation is not so easily achieved. In recent decades, encouraged by Western interest in oriental religions and philosophies, gurus, some qualified and some not, have been flourishing by pointing out the many pathways leading to the inner light. A few of them, mostly Indian and vastly experienced in the ways of yoga, are recognised as Masters of Prana, the yogic equivalent of Ch'i, the life-force to be drawn from the air around us. Charles Johnston, in his translation of *The Yoga Sutras of Patanjali, the Book of the Spiritual Man* (Stuart & Watkins, London, 1970), clearly describes the three limbs of yoga: concentration, meditation and contemplation:

> *The binding of the perceiving consciousness to a certain region is attention [concentration]; a holding of the perceiving consciousness in that region is meditation; when the perceiving consciousness in this meditation is wholly given to illuminating the essential meaning of the object contemplated and is freed from the sense of separateness and personality, this is contemplation.*

It is a great pity that meditation and, in fact, most forms of spiritual reflection are so unattainable to the average person who is in greatest need yet furthest from its fulfilment. Successful meditation is probably the most elusive of all 'self-help' methods. In spite of the countless volumes, increasing interest, qualified classes and courses, it remains a mystery far too complex to be learnt from the pages of a book.

And yet, you can walk into any health store or bookshop today and spend an indecisive hour searching through scores of titles on meditation and every other aspect of human improvement. Think of something you don't know about healthy, happy living and you'll find it on the rack. How to bring up your kids, how to tolerate your parents, how to make love, masturbate, increase your libido, grow new hair, face ageing and death with dignity, sleep soundly, relax and stop yourself from going crazy.

Much of the information is concerned with how to challenge and overcome the demon, stress. Anxiety and fear, resulting in depression and perhaps serious mental illness, have become as everyday and hard to cure as the common cold or bunion. Billions of dollars are spent each year on millions of multicoloured capsules containing temporary relief from the effects of daily doses of stress. Some of them help but none of them cure. And so, meditation in its many forms, both physic and mystic, has finally found its way from the East and taken a prominent place in the present and future of the West.

As serious and difficult as the search for religious faith, meditation is perhaps the most elusive of all pursuits leading towards peace of mind. Its results are the hardest of all to achieve, and will only come to the serious student through discipline and self-control far beyond the ordinary.

In spite of generous men like Yogi Ramacharaka, Patanjali and others, the true gurus of the inner self do not give away their knowledge lightly. Most of the information available is either a second-hand version from a Western enthusiast or the work of a renegade sensationalist from the Orient out to make a name for himself. Fame and fortune have no place in true meditation. It is only the rare oracle, dedicated to the selfless elevation of the mortal soul, who is qualified to teach another human being to meditate upon life and his or her place in it.

Does meditation have a place in the practice of Pa Tuan Tsin? Yes, it does. Simple initiation into forms of mind relaxation are taught in the second year at Chin Wu. It is stressed that progressive stages are only introduced to the advanced student and even then with great care and consideration. Masters of Chin Wu believe that indiscriminate dabbling can not only have the opposite effect to quietude, but may prove harmful. They go out of their way to lead into it with the utmost care, encouraging certain minds while gently suggesting infinite patience to others. After all, they say 'a bamboo door can believe it is a wooden door and never know the truth', which is a way of saying 'you don't have to come to terms with yourself ... millions don't and manage to get through life quite well'.

Any serious program of health improvement in today's anxiety-stricken environment would seem inadequate without at least a mention of meditation.

Contrary to many casual interpretations of meditation, it is not intended as a means of escaping reality or dulling the awareness of things that you would prefer to ignore or forget. It is an often difficult but always rewarding attempt to train and tune the mind, much as an athlete masters and disciplines the body. The end result of successful meditation is to increase one's awareness rather than diminish it and to transcend the painful and negative aspects of everyday life with serenity and greater efficiency.

Saint Theresa of Avila is said to have likened the human mind to an 'unbroken horse that would go anywhere except where you wanted it to'. Plato had a very original answer to the problems of a mind adrift. He compared it to a sailing ship commanded by a mutinous crew. With the true captain and his navigator safely in irons, the 'free' sailors take turns in steering the ship without knowledge or direction, foundering on the rocks or being hopelessly lost in strange oceans. Man's quest, he said, was to quell the mutiny, release the captain and navigator, plot a fresh but definite course and stay on it until the ultimate destination is reached.

A similar analogy is shown in these lines from a Sanskrit poem written in India between the second and fifth centuries BC:

The Wind turns a ship from its course upon the waters.
The wandering winds of the senses cast man's mind adrift,
and turn his better judgement from its courses.
When a man can still his senses I call him illumined.

Such pearls of wisdom are all very well, you may say, but how do I attain it? Where do I begin? One effective way of testing your powers of concentration is in 'counting your breath'. It may sound absurdly simple, but after trying it for fifteen minutes we realise how right Saint Theresa was and how close to the mark Plato's ship is sailing.

To find out for yourself, just stand, sit or lie in a comfortable position, in a spot with as little distraction as possible, and remain still. Begin counting each steady inhalation from one to eight and then begin again at one and so on for up to fifteen minutes. If nothing more, the exercise will give you an inkling of what if feels like to meditate and it will almost certainly alarm you to find how undisciplined your thoughts really are.

Although enough books and self-styled experts are available on the practices and philosophies of transcendentalism and yoga, for most of us simple methods of relaxing the mind will have to be enough. One such method was taught to me by Mr Wu. I had learned in lectures at Chin Wu that meditation had played a vital part in the lives of great Masters of the past. Only the simplest and most basic forms were taught to the novice, to be developed until years of practice brought their own reward. I visited Mr Wu unexpectedly one evening. He was not in the pool or on the terrace and his servant seemed unwilling to tell me where he was.

The servant bowed me to my usual chair and would have left to fix me a calamansi had I not insisted on knowing the whereabouts of his master. 'He is thinking, sir. You must find him quietly.' He pointed to a far corner of the garden which I had always believed to be a dense thicket of bamboo.

I found a cave-like opening in the ivory-smooth trunks. They creaked like the masts of a ship. The carpet of leaves made it possible to approach softly and the rustling all around deadened any noise I may have made. In the middle of the thicket was a clearing, in the centre of the clearing a small pool fed by a primitive tip-up fountain of the type found in Japanese monasteries. I saw the flash of carp in the pool, lit by the shards of moonlight that found their way into this hidden glade. They also lit a small shrine which the silent water surrounded. The air was heavy with incense from the cherry red sparks of joss sticks that pricked the dark before the shrine.

'Sit. I will tell you a poem and show you how to think about it.'

The quiet voice of Mr Wu came from the shadows. He sat naked to the waist, in the half lotus position, straight-backed and with the right hand resting in the left palm. His head was erect and facing the flowering joss, their tiny glow tinting the shrine. I copied his position and waited.

'You must concentrate on the burning tip of the joss through half-closed eyes. Clear your mind of all else but the depths. Listen to these words and try to memorise them. Think of nothing else. The words are from the Tao.

Close your eyes and you will see clearly.
Cease to listen and you will hear truth.
Be silent and your heart will sing.
Seek no contacts and you will find union.
Be still and you will move forward on the tide of spirit.
Be gentle and you will need no strength.
Be patient and you will achieve all things.
Be humble and you will remain entire.

In time I did memorise the words and forced myself to reflect on them. I learned to meditate to the best of my ability but soon I found my mind insisted on going its own way. The Taoist poem was meaningful but I had not been there. It was someone else's haven. I found that my basic concept of meditation was a sort of return to childhood. I had havens of my own. Most of us will admit that our appreciation of beautiful things, our absolute delight with the gifts of nature, has never been as clear-cut, as simply enchanting as when we are tiny. Perhaps it was because we knew so little and expected less. Can we remember our first serious contemplation of dew, those silver beads, strung diamond-brilliant along the network of a cobweb, the world reflected on a grass-tip or cradled by a leaf? Have flowers been as carefully scrutinised, their scents as openly breathed since then? Haven't trees lost a little of their majesty and skies become a little smaller? Are animals and insects half as friendly?

Even the harshest childhood had its vital moments, its magnificent discoveries, never to be recaptured but only to be looked back on as dreams. For me there were two such 'secrets'. They were places, sanctuaries known only to me. One was the great, rough arms of a giant elm, access gained by barked shins, grazed knees and no little risk of breaking my neck. Above, the wind-ruffled intricacy of leaves and birds; the darting light was like a cut-glass chandelier. The safe smell of moss and fungus, out of reach from everyone but God, whom I fervently believed was somewhere in that tree.

The other was in a field adjoining the school, which I was too young to attend. In summer its breezy grasses were uncut because no haymaker seemed to own it. Only the brewer's dray horse, great, brown and alone, stayed close to its hedges and explored it with his teeth. I found a spot where the cow parsley grew to the height of trees and the thick green clumps of dock leaves served as skating rinks for snails. There was an alder against an old brick wall and old, red dust came off when I leaned against it. I made a hiding place there, flattening the grass the way an animal does by turning round and round before lying down. For it I could watch the world, unseen except for clouds that moved over the wall and the sweet-scented wall-flowers that blew on top of it, with a lark above them. I shared that sacred spot with green-backed grasshoppers, scarlet ladybirds and a family of blackbirds that argued in the alder.

I was probably four years old at the time and yet I have learned to revisit those exclusive places of mine, so many years later. I can quite easily recall the rustle of the leaves that seemed to separate the sky, the piping of a visiting thrush and the smell of moss and fungus close to my cheek. It is not hard, if I concentrate, to clearly breathe the unmistakable perfume of red and yellow wallflowers and hear grass-hoppers shrilling all around me.

I chose those places to meditate because I am sure I was nearest to myself and to my Maker when I was there. Think back, if you intend to meditate, as far as you can go. Find the time and place where life was best and your world at its simplest, and begin again for those few moments.

An hour or two before retiring, go to the place of your choice. If it is in the spot where you practise Pa Tuan Tsin, so much the better. Set a lighted joss stick or candle in a small jar or other suitable container on the floor and turn out the light. Sit in the half lotus position, straighten the back and remain as erect as possible. Place the back of the relaxed right hand into the cupped palm of the relaxed left hand (like a swallow in its nest). Half close the eyes and concentrate intensely upon the red spark before you. Transfer any unwanted thoughts to the spark which for these moments has become your universe.

If the mind refuses to empty itself, recite the words of the poem (or any other which for you may have a pleasant meaning) and concentrate on your chosen time and place until a single element, a sight or sound or scent, perhaps all three, is floating there inside the flame. The essence of peace. Hold it there for five to fifteen minutes. If at first discomfort makes it difficult to remain perfectly still, try to ignore it: one aspect of meditation is endurance. If you can ignore pain for some seconds it will begin to be of less importance … eventually it will cease to exist.

The ultimate meditation is a trance-like state which leads to the ultimate control of bodily sensations. It is why the shaman, the fakir or the yogi can piece his own flesh without reaction and endure days, months or years of intense privation without a murmur.

Extend the period of meditation as you feel inclined, do not force yourself past a stage which commonsense warns is enough. Let it come slowly and do not expect it to come at all.

Sweet is solitude and peace of mind.
Sweet is to be free from fear or desire.
Hold fast to the truth as your refuge.

Gautama Buddha

THE POWER OF CH'I

The three walks of life;
to walk in the heavens,
to walk on the water,
but first to walk the way of the Tao

Lin Tui

PART
TWELVE

THE POWER OF CH'I

Reading back through these pages, I have tried to see if I have missed anything of importance to someone who is ready to begin improving his or her health through Pa Tuan Tsin. There are one or two points worth mentioning and a couple worth repeating.

I think the most important subject, which perhaps has not emerged as strongly as it should, is that of mental attitude. Firstly, admit that you are not as well as you could be and that unless you do something about it not only will you get no better, but eventually you will get worse. Secondly, it is important to be more than moderately interested in what you have read and more than tentative about trying it out. You should be utterly convinced by it and find the determination to practise it with the patience and fortitude any such intrusive procedure initially demands.

Since the message of this book is primarily aimed at people for whom, either through illness or advancing age, the bloom of youth as passed, this closing chapter is addressed to them in particular.

I wish I could have been even more persuasive, or found some unique way of making certain that you practise what I have suggested as religiously as I did not at least a month. If you were to do that I know you would continue until these exercises become as much a comforting part of your life as they are of mine. You will have experienced, whatever age you have reached, the wonderful changes that improved health can bring about through the simple process of concentrating on your breathing for a given period each day. You will have taken this blessing from the air around you. Air, Ch'i, Prana, Ki, intrinsic energy, life force, call it what you will, it is yours by right ... the first thing given to you on this earth and the last thing to be taken away.

Improving your health, the quality of your life and your attitude towards it, brings not only renewed confidence in yourself and your own capabilities, but a fresh confidence in life itself. The things that you find difficult to cope with at home or at work, the innermost worries that are yours and no one else's, even the people you prefer to avoid, will be more easily faced and overcome.

What then are the sorts of attitudes that may prevent you from taking full advantage of Pa Tuan Tsin? One is the fact that you may be fully aware of the need for exercise and already engaged in a full routine. Well, if this the case, whatever you are doing it obviously isn't enough or you would not have picked up this book. Any exercise is good but very few routines are benefiting us all-round, that is to say, as good for all of the inside as it is for all of the outside. As we have said, the Western concept of exercise tends to be cosmetic. As long as we develop good muscles, retain our shape and keep our waist as slim as we can, we look great and all is well.

We have made it very easy for ourselves to keep in good shape with every facility within easy reach of anyone with the need and energy to use it. We are constantly reminded of just how easy it is to keep looking well. If we don't have a swimming pool or tennis courts in our garden there are bound to be some within easy reach. We are constantly reminded of keep-fit programs that go hand in hand with certain breakfast cereals, easily practised in the privacy of our own room for as little as three minutes and a few cents a day. Television commercials, print ads and radio jingles offer us equipment we can buy or hire to row, pedal, push or pull towards a body like the one in the advertisement. We can have our hair dyed or even transplanted, our teeth capped, breasts inflated, noses changed, wrinkles removed, faces lifted and flesh shifted or carved off. There is nothing we cannot and will not do about our *outward* appearance while most of us let the *inside* upon which everything else depends, take care of itself and do very little to encourage it.

The Chinese, on the other hand (and many Asians, for that matter), consider the outward appearance of little importance compared to the inner condition. They have a saying which, loosely translated, means: 'It is useless to look forty when you are fifty, if inside you are sixty.' They also feel strongly about over-exercising certain parts of the body while neglecting other parts. As always, they have a saying: 'The legs of a bull will not get far on the heart of a chicken'. Or, 'A powerful arm does nothing for a weak stomach.'

'The world has always been quoted such fortune cookie philosophies,' you say, 'but what does it mean?' Well, it is true that in recent years Western medical science has taken another look at certain aspects of our physical culture. For instance, they have found that jogging for people of certain age, weight and condition can do far more harm than good, particularly jogging on concrete, which has a jarring effect on the spine and may have serious repercussions in later years. The rigours of the weight-lifting gym can do more harm than good unless carefully overseen. Even the beneficial rays of the sun have come under increasing scrutiny with the realisation that indiscriminate sunbathing when young not only ages skin long before its time, but result in skin disease and even cancer later on. On the other hand, health programs, exercise methods, preventive medicine, mythical cures from the Orient, and so on, are getting more and more attention from occidental experts. 'Acupuncture, moxibustion, herb remedies, youth drugs, love philtres and massage, are age-old healing methods that astound modern medical science', was one remark made by leading American surgeon, Dr Samuel Rosen, on his return from China in 1970. He had been invited to witness acupuncture and other practices of Chinese folk medicine. He summed up for the *New York Times* as follows: 'I have seen the past and it works'.

For thousands of years strict followers of Yoga, Zen, other Asian and some African cults have been able to influence such functions as pulse rate, breathing, digestion, sexual control, metabolism and kidney activity at will. They can slow the heartbeat to what would normally be lethal levels, reduce their respiration to one breath every few minutes and suspend the life force to enable themselves to be buried alive for days. They have total control of the reflexes that cause normal people to avoid intense pain and can divert them at will, allowing spikes and blades to pierce their flesh without causing the slightest reaction, even controlling the flow of blood.

Why should we disbelieve, then, astounding claims of longevity or question such feats as those accomplished by the 'mountain leapers' of Tibet. These monks who live in rugged and almost inaccessible upland wastes long ago produced their own version of 'bionic man'. By practising the art of Lung-gom they are able to cover the ground in great leaps and bounds, bouncing from one spot to the next with the elasticity of an India Rubber ball. They have been known to cover a distance of 480 kilometres between sunrise of one day and midday of the next, travelling at a speed of 16 kilometres per hour over very inhospitable terrain. Great marathon runners average 19 kilometres per hour on good roads for a maximum of two hours at a stretch.

Another classic example is the Tibetan practice of Tumo, the art of bearing the cold. Through a highly complex system of breathing exercises and meditation these hermits are able to live high up in the regions of permanent snow and go about completely naked or in nothing but a thin cotton garment. The test of a novice would be enough to kill any other human being; after months of bathing in icy streams and sitting naked in the snow, he is wrapped in a sheet which has been dipped through a hole in the ice of a lake, and left to sit outside all night. The sheet must be completely dried by his body heat and replaced by a wet one at least three times before sunrise.

Of course, such superhuman accomplishments don't come easily. A lifetime of self-discipline leads to an ordeal such as the training for Lung-gom, where the initiate must sit in complete darkness and seclusion for thirty-nine months, all the while performing deep-breathing exercises. Is such dedication to developing the human body, mind and soul to such limits any less valuable than spending billions to build a false one?

A question I am often asked, and something about which you may be wondering, is what of the quality of air? 'What use is it,' you may ask, 'for me to apply myself to this business of breathing properly when I live in a city where the air is so foul I would be wiser breathing as little of it as possible?' We have lived with pollution and its ever-present threats for too long not to be aware of the difference between good and bad air. Of course, one who daily breathes the untainted air of high altitudes, of the open countryside or of the sea, is more fortunate than one who has to make the best of city smog. It even 'tastes' better.

THE AIR WE BREATHE

Fortunately, nature has equipped every one of us with a built-in filtering and refining system which, provided we use it properly, renders even the worst air breathable, as long as there is sufficient oxygen present. What is meant by using it properly? The answer is simple. By *always* inhaling through the nose and *never* inhaling through the mouth. Again, the Chinese have a saying: 'Only a fool will stuff food up his nose. To take air through the mouth is no better.' Not as absurd as it sounds, it simply demonstrates that the nostrils are intended for breathing and the mouth is intended for eating.

A more recent, and perhaps more practical, illustration is found in 'The Good Health Battle Plan' by Dr Donald Norfolk, published in *Cosmopolitan*.

One habit to be avoided is mouth-breathing. When we breathe though the nose, we warm and filter the inspired air. It has been estimated that we inhale 20 billion particles of foreign matter a day. When we breathe through the nose, most of these bits of dirt and dust are trapped in the sticky mucus that lines the airways. From there they are wafted harmlessly to the stomach by the cilia, the fine hairs that exert a constant sweeping action over the surface of the mucus membranes. Experimental animals have been given dirty air to breathe at temperatures ranging from 500°C to minus 100°C and in every case, the air was cleaned and warmed to body temperature before it entered the lungs. Such is the efficiency of the body's air-conditioning apparatus, providing it is not by-passed by breathing through the mouth. A further advantage of breathing through the nose is that it helps clear the sinuses.

The other thing we can do to make the most of our share of oxygen is to let it in, not shut it out. Ventilation is as sensible as breathing through the apparatus we have been given for the purpose. We know that if we shut ourselves in a confined space for long enough, we will use up the oxygen and continually recycle the air until it becomes nothing but waste, as used up and useless as any other of the body's waste matters.

For those who live in cold climates the houses, places of work and, particularly, bedrooms, are too often tightly sealed for the sake of our health. We are led to believe that cold is bad for us and that exposure to it can lead to colds, flu and other serious bronchial and respiratory illnesses. Of course, it can if we allow the temperature to drop too low, or wear inadequate clothing and have insufficient covering on our beds. But we were meant to live with cold, and living with it intelligently is not difficult.

The same applies to those who live in the tropics. Air-conditioning, which depends on sealed space for efficiency, is a poor alternative to fresh air, no matter how high its temperature. The problem of keeping cool is generally greater for Western people living in Eastern climates. No matter how long a European lives in an equatorial or excessively hot country, most find it difficult to survive comfortably without air-conditioning. In the days of the Raj, in the furnace heat of India, the sahibs and memsahibs turned to punkah fans and hill stations for relief. Now many Europeans pay mightily for full air-conditioned hotels, accommodation and offices while the natives of that country continue to live and work in the conditions they were born in.

The air we breathe is made up of positive (destructive) ions, and negative (energy-giving) ions. The less oxygen or pure air in our surroundings the more prevalent the positive ions; the more oxygen or pure air in our surroundings, the more prevalent the negative ions. That is to say, the rarefied air of a mountain top, the middle of a forest or a field, with its oxygen-making foliage and plant life, or the ozone of an ocean, would be predominantly made up of life-giving negative ions. The further we get away from these natural ideals and the closer to cities, with their industrial complexes, traffic and lack of greenery, the more laden the air becomes with unhealthy positive ions.

The problem is considered serious by many scientists. The study of biometeorology, which has been taking place since the 1930s, is of major importance in such countries as Switzerland, East Germany and Hungary, and was best summed up in *The Ion Effect* (Fred Sokya and Alan Edmonds, Bantam, New York, 1978). Soyka, who spent many years researching his subject throughout the world, explains how air electricity rules our lives and health. He analyses the adverse effects of those bizarre climatic conditions known as the 'Witches' Winds'; the Föhn of the European Alps; Italy's sirocco; the Santa Ana in California, known to the Indians as the 'Bitter Winds', which blows from the deserts of northern Arizona down into Mexico; the Chinook of Western Canada and the United States; the Sharav (or Hamsin) of Israel and the Middle East; and the sinister Mistral of southern France. All of these winds have strange and disquieting effects upon those in their path. Suicide rates roar, traffic accidents become almost epidemic and, at best, we feel a little 'under the weather' or 'out of sorts'.

The significant thing about these observations seems to be that the air during these winds is found to be predominantly charged with positive ions and very low on negative ions, similar to the conditions we have created in our cities and modern buildings through air-conditioning and central heating — not to mention the pollution of transportation and industry.

These discoveries led some of the world's most eminent scientists to turn their attention to the development of ionisation in the 1970s. Dr Albert P. Kreuper, Emeritus Professor of Bacteriology at the University of California, and Israel's Dr Felix Gad Sulman put up a case so convincing that the World Health Organisation and World Meteorological Organisation cooperated in drawing such environmental dangers to the notice of architects and town planners, car and aircraft designers, and others who create the environments that most of us are forced to live with.

Russia and the nations of eastern Europe are far more advanced in biometeorology than the nations of the West, with the exception of Switzerland. In these countries, ionisers are a part of standard hospital equipment in operating theatres, post-operative recovery wards, delivery rooms and intensive care units. (Ionisers are electronic units that emit negative ions.)

In 1975, an Eastern German doctor treated more than 11 000 patients with 'neg-ion' therapy. Brazilian hospitals have long been using ion generators, and Switzerland's Dr Russel Stark initiated its use in factories and office complexes with a dramatic improvement in staff performance.

CH'I — THE POWER WITHIN!

I suppose the most pointed, and certainly the most frequent, question I am asked in relation to my faith in the cultivation of Ch'i is, 'What makes you so positive about the effects of these breathing exercises? Surely any form of exercise, considering the fact that you were out of condition at the time, would have made you look and feel better. Do you really think it is worth putting into a book?'

Perhaps then, this the best question with which to conclude.

My belief in the power of Ch'i or, to sound less dramatic, the absolute importance of developing any degree of inner strength through breath control, was, of course, given to me by personal acquaintance with the Chin Wu School. In the early stages, I was impressed and awed by the everyday displays of sheer physical excellence that I saw there. Then this astonishment grew into genuine interest and complete enthusiasm. The infinite patience and flawless example of remarkable people — like Mr Wu, Master Chan, Johnny Cheutin, the White Crane champion I have called 'D', and so many other students and instructors of Wu Shu — cannot fail to persuade even the most stubborn cynic. To witness and become even a small part of such power coupled with humility is in itself a revelation. But I also think it was the sheer commonsense of Chin Wu philosophy, the practical concept of breathing for health that convinced me and provided the discipline.

I considered my own background. I remembered how, when physical effort had been my way of life, I had relied on the ability to breathe properly as a matter of course; I used breath as a tool to not only accomplish manual labour but to actually enjoy it. I remember that it would have been impossible to fell a tree without breathing being an integral part of bodily rhythm; to try to swing an axe or a hammer all day without the measured lung power to drive home force would be futile.

I then realised, with a measure of shock, that since I had given up the physical, outdoor life and begun the long climb to respectability, responsibility and 'success', I had also given up the ability to breathe. It came to me that in almost a quarter of a century I had forgotten what real breathing was like. I reflected upon the years of sitting behind a desk, the wheel of a car, in an easy chair before a television screen, never conscious of my breath unless I was forced to use it, and only to find myself 'out of it' in a matter of minutes.

Although I have tried to pass on as effectively as possible the way I feel about breathing for health, I fully realise that the personal experiences and convictions of one person are rarely enough to motivate another. Nevertheless, it may be worth relating what is perhaps the closest to tangible proof of the power of Ch'i.

Although I had fallen into the trap of 'good living' and experiencing the gradual physical decline that so often goes with it, I had never been really ill. I had not seen the inside of a hospital and seldom called upon a doctor, even at the age of forty-five. I had all my own teeth, a good head of hair and had always been strong, due perhaps to so many years of healthy physical work in my younger days. But, although I had survived the stresses and strains of a 'busy' life as best I could, it had left me a fairly heavy drinker and an even heavier smoker. Only when my stamina was suddenly tried did it occur to me that I had been deceiving myself for a long time.

Then in March 1975, whilst living in the Philippines, I began to lose my voice. I put it down to the epidemic of laryngitis that was going around Manila at the time and, apart from inhaling various concoctions and resting my voice when possible, I waited without too much concern for it to pass.

I was nearing the end of my first year with Chin Wu and on one particular evening I had been called upon to lead the class through the warm-up exercises and Pa Tuan Tsin. It was customary to count loudly for each set of movements and when my voice failed completely in the middle of a set Master C. called a replacement and led me into his little office.

'Have you seen a doctor about your throat?' he asked, casually. I nodded. 'What does he say?' 'Laryngitis,' I croaked. 'Would you come to see a Chinese doctor?' His tone was so serious and his eyes so steady that I quickly agreed.

The man he took me to could have been a grocer or a retired gardener. Instead, he was one of the most famous traditional Chinese doctors in the Philippines. He sat me down and looked me over almost nonchalantly, as though appraising my clothes. Without a word, he left the small table that served as his desk and stood before me. 'Take off your shoes and shirt and breathe quietly,' he said, and he put his fingertips very lightly on the soles of my feet, my ankles, my underarms and my neck and throat. At each point of contact he paused for up to ten or twenty seconds, his eyes closed and raised to the ceiling. In less than a minute he had finished his examination and, after a short discussion with Master C., he bowed us out.

'He says you have a growth on the larynx,' Master C. said briskly as soon as we were outside. 'He says you must tell your doctor to check you into the hospital for a biopsy without delay. It has been with you for months.'

The shock of a positive cancer test is probably one of the most severe emotions one can face. It is an overwhelming feeling of lonely despair coupled with a little flame of hope that usually flickers until it is put out. A feeling of having been singled out and punished. But it is not really something one can attempt to describe to another, so I will try no further. It is enough to say that in little more than forty-eight hours I was being fitted for my radiation mask in the Radiotherapy Unit of Hammersmith Hospital, just outside central London. The experiences and emotions that one goes through while undergoing radiotherapy is a subject that would fill another book and is certainly not necessary here. What is relevant is the way in which Pa Tuan Tsin helped me through five consecutive weeks of maximum super-voltage, its effect on the results of the treatment and the vital part it played in my rehabilitation.

A BBC interviewer asked me a rather obvious if not well thought out question. 'If,' said the confident woman, 'you were already a regular practitioner of the respiratory exercise routine you so enthusiastically recommend, when you detected so classic a respiratory disease did it not cast a little doubt upon the preventive powers the exercises claim to offer?'

It had of course, crossed my mind, until the Director of Radiotherapy, and one of Britain's leading specialists, explained that science can not detect when, why or where malignant cells first develop. In respiratory cancer (throat and lungs) it is firmly believed that heavy smoking, together with poor respiratory function considerably increases the grim prospect, but is not necessarily its root cause. Some people, he explained, may have given up smoking for years and still suffer from the disease, the seeds of which can have been sown up to twenty years earlier. Once there and once activated it must be fought with all the power of the universe and the mortal soul. The BBC journalist seemed little impressed by this answer, as she mashed out another half-smoked cigarette among the thirty or forty already in the ashtray beside her.

The first days of treatment are briefly described in my diary:

THE VICARAGE. MAY 16TH. 6.30 A.M.

We are staying the weekend at the Vicarage. It is in a lovely old place about thirty minutes from Waterloo. This lovely part, which is on a green, slow-flowing river hidden by willows has become a little hemmed-in by housing estates, but there are some things they cannot ruin and this river is one of them. Tomorrow is my first day of treatment. My first dose of radiation, then there are only twenty-nine to go. The doc says thirty doses are as far as they can go without risk of permanent damage. My mask is finished and fits like a skin. The planning is done and the calculations that will direct the beam have been checked and rechecked and entered in a thin record book with my name on it. Tomorrow the fight begins. I think of all the times I have complained and all the times I have almost given up. And I tell you, God, I am ashamed. The water of that river is calm and deep. Its current is sluggish and ripples round the stems of lilies. Dragonflies patrol the clumps of reeds and a family of ducks wades among them to head upstream. It is dawn and I have come here to take my breathing exercises and practise the dance of the Mantis. I tried doing it in the Vicarage garden but the sight of it alarmed the neighbours. I wonder how the Shaolin monks handled cancer.

St James Park. May 17th. 6 a.m.

The first morning of my treatment begins as bravely as a warrior preparing for combat. I jog to St. James Park to single out my favourite tree. It is 6 a.m. and grey, as I bounce past faces black, brown, cream and yellow. I feel like waving to the pink ones. Past the thronging bus stops, crowds poised at pedestrian crossings like United Nations assault troops waiting for a signal. I want to wave to them all. 'Morning' all ... 'ave a nice day, we're all English now ... it's us against the rest.' They seem to know I'm a stranger. Skipping over a dog poop, nimble as a forty-seven-year-old gnome. I want to shout at them. 'I belong here y'know. Born and bred. In uniform at fourteen, me. I've got a right to be here. This is my country.' The faces don't encourage such frivolity.

In the park, among exploding buds and under spreads of new green, a golden ash vibrating in the breeze; gleaming chestnut flanks trot and canter along the bridle paths. Immaculate riders, some uniformed in the regimental blue of Guards, others sport the tailored habit and hard hat of the very rich. A tramp rolls from under a shelter of dew-damp reck chairs; they are propped against a fallen elm ... the elm had taken a century or to two to grow, now its heart is eaten out with elm blight all the way from Holland. The tramp adjusts the newspaper beneath his coat, much as a passing lady rider adjusts her silken cravat, and settles down to watch me approach the bottom of my imaginary mountain.

The radiation tank. May 18th.

Half a ton of lead shifts aside like a Church tank cranking its turret onto a feeble target. I feel like a grain of sand, singled out from a desert. All the power of the universe is aimed at my throat. That great clink, the nippy little nurse had told me before retreating in her soft white shoes, was the lead shielding sliding aside, to let the weasel see the rabbit. I resented her. Untouchable in her neat early morning white, smelling of starch and Lifebuoy as she bends close to bolt the protective shield in place, warm breath, faintly Pepsodent. Where's the mumsy one with her 'cuppa and Woodbine' manner?

'Try not to swallow and whatever happens don't move.' Move? How can I move? With this thing holding me from chin to chest like a vice. I feel like Frankenstein's dangerous puppet. My eyes swivel to the Mobiltron poised above me, bit as a searchlight. The Mobiltron, invention of the great and humane, clanked around on its giant crane arm. Tiny window in its middle winking like a cyclop's eye, fine, crossed hairs sighting its centre. Power of a thousand suns. That's what the Japs had said when the Yanks dropped it on Hiroshima. Baked thousands of people in their

*tracks and scorched the world. Now here it was, tame as a working
elephant. Trundling obediently on its chain around this giant's quadrant
to try and save another life.*

*'You won't feel anything,' she had said as she adjusted the wedge under
my arched back. 'Just a sort of thump as the lead drops then a faint
buzzing.' She smiled briefly as a blink. 'Larynx is easy to get at. Only
two minutes each side. Try to think of something else.' I thought of my
spot under the alder and the sound of flies buzzing on the wall, a ladybird
climbing a stalk of grass. And the buzz of the Mobiltron became a bright
green grasshopper rubbing its back legs together.*

Throughout the five weeks of super-voltage radiation, the early
morning practise of Pa Tuan Tsin was not only a great source of
physical and mental wellbeing but it produced tangible and
somewhat amazing results. Exposure to intense radiation is expected
to have its negative side-effects, and each patient is given a little book
to warn and prepare them for what is to come. Weight loss, loss of
appetite, loss of sleep and a general downturn in spirit are the most
typical. I am glad to say that at no time did I experience any of these.
I slept soundly without sedatives, ate ravenously, drank my quota of
draught Guinness at the 'local' each evening and maintained a steady
certainty about the outcome.

Even case-hardened doctors and nurses were impressed and
asked me to demonstrate the Precious Set of Eight. It was their
interest and obvious understanding of the importance of respiratory
exercise that prompted me to write and publish what had been given
to me.

Before leaving you to decide whether you will add this book to
those on the shelf to be dusted once a week, or whether you will open
it each morning and begin improving your health, there is one brief
point I feel I must repeat. While compiling this material, I have
tussled with the nagging concern that, in spite of my efforts to
explain to the contrary, the result may be misinterpreted as an
attempt to reach or preach some facets of the marital arts. I feel I
must, for the last time, emphasise that it is not. In presenting a little of
the history of Wu Shu and mentioning a few of its past and present
champions, I have merely tried to provide a background to the
exercises that are the book's only purpose. It only represents that
which I have learned and used to my great benefit from the Chin Wu
Athletic Association of the Philippines, those connected with it, and
in particular Master Shakespeare Chan who gave me permission to
pass it on in this way.

Any serious student of Wu Shu or any other form of marital art would probably consider it the ABC of their craft. Although they may not have been fully aware of the ancient Shaolin ritual of Pa Tuan Tsin they would certainly have grounded their training on some similar routine of breathing exercises, and may consider it tame reading indeed. One cannot be involved in Wu Shu without being humbly aware of the tremendous physical, mental and material demands made upon the genuine follower who hopes for a recognised place in this exceptional society. The rigid discipline of self-denial throughout the better part of a lifetime, the personal courage and individual conquest set the true believer aside from the ordinary.

It seems I have said all that I can about the importance of improved breathing and cultivation of the vital Ch'i through the Eight Precious Sets of Exercises. Even if they do not become a regular part of your daily life you may at least have faced the shape you are in and realised that any improvement in your breathing habits can only help you to live and love longer through the power of Ch'i. Proof? The real proof is within you. Only your own efforts and their results will prove to be of any real meaning or benefit to you: your own patience and your own fortitude. This book can only show you the foot of the mountain, it cannot make you climb.

For me the opportunity came later in my life than I would have liked and at a time when total dedication to the demands and disciplines were both impractical and impossible. It may well be the same for you. I have satisfied myself with knowledge enough to pass on in the interests of improved health and am grateful to my teachers and friends in the Brotherhood for the opportunity. The intricacies and refinements to be found further up the mountain I leave to those who have earned the right to teach it.

It is up to you how far you go or whether you turn back before you begin. It's your life, your spirit, your body and your health. Master Chee Soo sums it up with a saying passed on by his Master, Chan Lee: 'A reflection in a pool never reveals its depth. To know that, you must enter the water.' So, get your feet wet.

The yogis of old were right: in this competitive and demanding age, keeping fit and able is not just a fad, it is a duty. A duty to yourself, the one that gave you life and those who depend upon you to remain strong. Stop relying on those inadequate little breaths and start learning to fill your lungs the way you were intended to. Start breathing for your life and love. And when you have found what it can do for you, teach it to others so that we can all live longer and love longer through the power of Ch'i.

Where to Learn More About Therapeutic and Healing Chi Kung

If you follow the instructions in this book as carefully as you can, applying those aspects of it you feel most comfortable with through as much patience, tolerance and discipline as you can, you will feel immediate and surprising benefits. If you are able to preserve and create your own routine, those benefits will increase rapidly and after about six weeks of careful practice, plus the support of compatible exercise and diet, Chi Kung will have become a valuable part of your life. Whether you continue to apply it or allow it to become another passing fad is up to you — only you have the power to decide.

If you find yourself suited to breathing exercises and wish to learn more under qualified instruction look up martial arts instructors in the telephone book and make enquiries. Wherever you live, there is likely to be a Tai Chi or Kung Fu master who can advise you. In some Western countries there is the Choy Lee Fut Federation which is in direct association with the Therapeutic Chi Kung (Worldwide) China.

Choy Lee Fut Chi Kung, also known as 'Shaolin Lohan Chi Kung was passed down by the Shaolin Monk, Choy Fook to Chan Heung, the founder of Choy Lee Fut Kung Fu in the middle of last century. The word *Lohan* means 'Arhat' (the venerated one, the perfect being, from the language of Indian Yoga) — one who has realised the energising effects of 'stream-entry', the Buddhist expression for the origin of this ancient form of Chi Kung.

The form not only promotes health and fitness through mastery of the universal breath but also encourages realisation of 'The Wisdom' — intrinsic energy gained by the acceptance of Shunyata, the sublime state of nothingness or quietude. It also teaches a deep and abiding compassion towards all living things. It believes that our total wellbeing depends as much upon the condition of our emotions, or inner environment, as it does on our physical circumstances, or outer environment. The aim, as in all things Chinese, is to develop and maintain the correct balance between these opposing elements, through gaining control first of the external, the physical (body) then the internal, the metaphysical (mind and spirit). Let us call it self-discipline ... and we are back to the three passwords to achievement — Patience, Tolerance and Discipline.

The monk Choy Fook took advantage of the mountain retreat around the Temple of Shaolin as Tamo had done centuries before him. From the untamed terrain he took the ways of the wild, the survival techniques of the five animal forms — The Tiger, The Snake, The Crane, The Leopard, and the combined and mystical powers of The Dragon. He observed minutely their ways, their habits, their every movement and sound, combining what he learned with the human life force, the understanding and control of the breath. This he used to devise three precious sets of exercises.

1 *Lohan Kung* or 'Bodhidarma Lohan eighteen hands'. Eighteen carefully studied movements coupled with specific breathing exercises taken from the five animal forms designed to activate the flow of Ch'i. It is excellent for building and maintaining health and fitness, and protecting the body against attack. Among the graceful movements are exercises to combat physical and mental ailments such as high or low blood pressure, tension and stress-related conditions.

2 *Siu Lohan* or 'The Small Arhat'. With fewer movements the emphasis is more on control of the mind than the body. This form introduces sound as well as semi-meditational postures. It uses the powers of the mind (imagination, visualisation, contemplation) to generate Ch'i energy, rather than movement of the limbs. Remember the Tan T'ien can only be located through the will of the mind as explained on pages 73–75.

3 *Da Lohan* or 'The Big Arhat'. Again, a series of semi-meditational postures in various configurations, for example, the Horse and Bow Stances, sitting, lying down, full and half Lotus. Da Lohan promotes stillness or quietude through meditation. From the state of eternity all control is achieved through this pure and simple form of breathing exercise.

If you wish to obtain a video, made in conjunction with the book *Power of Chi*, contact the publisher of this book for details.

BIBLIOGRAPHY

Blofeld, John. *Taoism the Quest for Immortality*, Allen & Unwin/Mandala, UK, 1979.

Chang, E.C., translated by. *Knocking at the Gate of Life*, Thorsons, UK, 1986.

Chia, Mantak. *Awaken Health Energy Through the Tao*, Aurora Press, USA, 1983.

China Sports and New World Press, joint editors. *Traditional Chinese Fitness Exercises*, China, 1984.

Choy Lee Fut Federation. Lohan Kung — *Martial Fitness, Healing Art*, 1983.

Cooper, J.C. *Chinese Alchemy: The Taoist Quest for Immortality*, Aquarian Press, UK, 1984.

Deng Ming Dao. *The Wandering Daoist*, Harper & Row, USA, 1983.

Iijima, Reverend Kanjitsu. *Buddhist Yoga*, Japan, 1975.

Jwing-Ming, Dr Yang. *Chi Kung Health and Martial Arts*, Yang Martial Arts Academy, Boston, Massachusetts, 1985.

Jwing-Ming, Dr Yang. *Eight Pieces of Brocade, Chi Kung Exercises*, Yang Martial Arts Academy, Boston, Massachusetts, 1988.

Luk, Charles and Lu Kuan Yu. *Chinese Yoga, Taoist Alchemy*, Rider, USA, 1967.

Luk, Charles and Lu Kuan Yu. *The Secrets of Chinese Meditation*, Rider, USA, 1964.

Marks, Captain Tom. *Chinese Chin Kung for Physical and Mental Health*, Martial Arts Incorporated (distributed by McLisa Enterprises, Honolulu), Taipei, 1975.

Montaigue, Erle. *Self-healing Chinese Exercises for Health and Longevity*, Boobooks, Sydney, 1986.

Nakamura, Takashi. *Oriental Breathing Therapy*, Japan Publications Incorporated, Japan, 1981.

Pike, Geoff. *The Power of Ch'i*, Bay Books, Sydney, 1980.

Siou, Lily PhD and Tuttle, Charles E. *Chi Kung, Mastering the Unseen Life Force*, Rutland, Vermont, 1975.

Tohei, Koichi. *Book of Ki, Coordinating Mind and Body*, Japan Publications.

Tohei, Koichi and Ki No Kenkyuko. *Kiatsu, Ki Life Force*, Tokyo, 1983.

Wang Pei Sheng and Chen Guan Hua. *Relaxing and Calming Qigong*, Peace Book Co. and New World Press, China, 1986.

Zhang Ming Wu and Sun Xing Yuan, compiled by. *Chinese Qigong Therapy*, Shandon Science and Technology Press, China, 1985.

INDEX

A

abdominal exercises 113, 115, 118, 137, 236-44

Achilles tendon, stretch exercises for 188, 191

acupuncture 67-8

adductor stretch exercises 190, 192

aerobic dance 180-1

ageing 198-202, 254-6

air-conditioning 258

air pressure within the body 60-2

air quality 257-9

alcohol 78, 201, 235

alertness, exercises for 124

ankles, exercises for 120, 139

arms
exercises for 111-12, 116, 137, 141
testing flexibility of 20

aspirin 218

atherosclerosis 217

B

back
exercises for 113, 117, 118, 137
flexibility exercise 186

Back Cross Stance 105-6

bad breath 222

balance, exercises for 94, 97, 99-100, 103, 139

Bend Bamboo exercise 154-5

Bend Like the Grass exercise 167-8

bicycling 180-1

biometeorology 258-9

blood cleansers 218-19

blood pressure 221, 222

Bow Stance 97-8, 122

bread 235

breakfast 233

breathing
see also deep breathing; lungs
benefits of exercises 259-60
exercises 147-60; see also Chi Kung; Pa Tuan Tsin
importance of 54-66
patterns 57
testing 18-19

C

calorie content 234

calves
exercises for 139
stretch exercises for 188, 191

carbohydrates 230-1

Carradine, David 38, 46

carrots 235

Catch the Swallow exercise 158-9

Ch'ang Ming 209-11

channels of Ch'i 67-73

Chen Ch'i 60-1

chest, exercises for 116, 137

Ch'i
definition 11-12
explanation 54-66
Masters 45-52
meridians 67-73

Chi Kung
and ageing 198-202
basic exercises 86-91
benefit 67-8
and nutrition 205-16

Chin Wu
description 30-6
Masters 46-52
meditation 248

Chinese splits 195

Chinese Temple Boxing
see Wu Shu

Chiuten, Johnny 47-8

cholesterol 217-20
effect of exercise 178

circulation, exercises for 94, 107, 110

clothing for Pa Tuan Tsin 86

complete breathing see deep breathing

concentration 74-6
for Chi Kung 87
preparation exercises 107

Confucius 208

constipation, exercise to relieve 94

cookware 231

crash diets 221, 226

Crunches (exercise) 244

D

deep breathing
Chi Kung exercises 87-91
definition 59-60
first steps 19, 64-6

diet 77-9
combined with exercise 173-4
effect on ageing 201
nutrition and Chi Kung 205-35

diet diary 229-30

dieting for weight loss 221-35

digestion, exercise to aid 94

E

eating see diet

eggs 235

'Eight Precious Sets of Exercises' see Pa Tuan Tsin

enzymes 55

exercise 172-85
  choosing 175, 180-1
  duration of 179
  effect on ageing 202
  equipment 182
  for weight loss 223
  importance of 77, 78, 255
  starting 182-3
  walking 196-7
exercise bike 182
exercises
  see also stretching exercises
  abdominal 236-44
  advanced 161-71
  breathing 147-60
  Chi Kung breathing 86-91
  flexibility 183-6
  Pa Tuan Tsin 123-46
  stances 93-106
  warm-up 107-22
Eye of the Tiger exercise
  139-40

F

Face the Tiger exercise 153
fad diets 226
fat in diet 218
fatigue
  diet 222
  exercises to relieve 133
fattening foods 234
feet, exercises for 110, 139
fighting 37-8, 40-4
Finger Flicking exercise 109
fish 211
fish oil 219
fitness see physical fitness
'Five Flavours of Life' 211, 213
flavourings 211
flexibility
  see also stretching exercises
  exercises for 117, 186-95
  importance of 183-5
  testing 19-20

food *see* diet
food groups 229
foot channels 69
foot positions 93
foot shaking exercise 110
footwear for Pa Tuan Tsin 86
Front Cross Stance 103-4
fruit 213, 232
garlic 224-5
glucose 183
grains 213

G

Grip the Swallow's Egg
  exercise 141-3
groin stretch exercise 190
gum chewing 233
gyms 175-6

H

Half-knee Stance 101-2
hamstring stretch exercises
  188, 191
hand channels 69
hand-fighting 38
Hatha Yoga 178
Head Rolling exercise 108
'health' foods 224
heart
  cholesterol 217-20
  health 176, 178
heart attack prevention 220
High Snap Kick exercise 166
hip exercise 129
holistic healing 68, 208-9
Horse Stance 94-5
hypertension 221, 222

I

imagination 75
immune system during
  ageing 200
India 42

indigestion 222
injuries
  exercise to relieve 133
  sports 176-7
internal organs 60, 67, 68, 200
ionisation 259

J

Jeet Kune Do 45
jing 67
jogging 180=1
Judo 38

K

Karate 38
kelp 225
Kicking Shadows exercise 164
kicking techniques 164-6
kidneys, exercises for 115, 137
kilojoule content 234
kneecap 122
knees, exercises for 121
Kung Fu, Western popularity
  of 37-8, 55
  see also Wu Shu 41
Kuo Shu 41

L

lactic acid 183
Lao Tzu 208
Lee, Bruce 37-8, 44, 45-6
Lee, James 37
leg positions 93
legs
  see also calves
  exercises for 94, 97, 99-100,
    103, 111, 119, 129, 141
  stretching exercises for
    117, 118, 137, 162, 193
  testing flexibility 19-20
life span 199
Lift Iron Horse exercise 156=7
Lift the Rock exercise 135=6